ESSENTIAL
OILS
for Beauty, Wellness,
and the Home

ESSENTIAL OILS

for Beauty, Wellness, and the Home

100 Natural, Nontoxic Recipes for the Beginner and Beyond

ALICIA ATKINSON

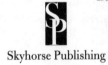

Skyhorse Publishing

Skyhorse Publishing books may be purchased in bulk at special discounts for sales promotion, corporate gifts, fund-raising, or educational purposes. Special editions can also be created to specifications. For details, contact the Special Sales Department, Skyhorse Publishing, 307 West 36th Street, 11th Floor, New York, NY 10018 or info@skyhorsepublishing.com.

Skyhorse® and Skyhorse Publishing® are registered trademarks of Skyhorse Publishing, Inc.®, a Delaware corporation.

Visit our website at www.skyhorsepublishing.com.

10 9 8 7 6 5 4 3 2 1

Library of Congress Cataloging-in-Publication Data is available on file.

Cover design by Jane Sheppard
Cover photo credit: iStock Photography

Print ISBN: 978–1–63450–495-9
Ebook ISBN: 978–1–5107–0161-8

Printed in the United States of America

Contents

PART ONE
Introduction to Essential Oils

WHAT ARE ESSENTIAL OILS?

The simplest way to describe essential oils is by their function: essential oils are essentially a plant's own medicine and communication system. They help plants ward off disease and invaders, and to heal themselves when they get damaged. Essential oils also allow plants to attract animals that help plants with pollination. Essential oils exist within the leaves, flowers, stems, roots, berries, resin, and bark of plants.

Scientifically, essential oils are complex secondary metabolites. This means, they are not the building blocks of the plant such as proteins and carbohydrates, but are made by the plant for its benefit. Secondary metabolites do not feed the plants, nor are they mandatory for their daily survival. However, secondary metabolites have developed to increase the long-term survival of individual plants and their species as a whole. Secondary metabolites are unique to certain plant groups as opposed to primary metabolites that are found in all plant species. Besides aromatic essential oils, a common secondary metabolite is pigmentation. Pigments attract or repel animals, as well as protect plants from sun damage and fruits from spoilage. Essential oils also perform these functions and many others.

Essential oils are also not singular compounds; they are instead a mixture of many, many chemical constituents that work together to benefit the plant. While each compound itself has certain benefits, the essential oil as a whole is more effective than the individual compounds. This synergistic effect also takes place between different essential oils when they are used in combination. Gas spectrometers are often used to break essential oils down to assess their individual compounds. The names of many of these compounds are listed with the most common essential oils in this book, but there are certain types of compounds that are found in most essential oils. The most prevalent compounds in essential oils are terpenes, which are hydrocarbon molecules with a different amounts of hydrogen atoms (which give them their classifications), but always ten carbon atoms. Other compounds and molecules commonly found in essential oils include alcohols, aldehydes, ethers, ketones, alkaloids, and acids.

In order to retrieve these compounds and use them beneficially for humans, we either cold-press them out of rinds or flowers, use solvents to extract them, or most commonly, we use steam distillation to retrieve them.

These processes purify the essential oils, also known as essence oils or volatile oils, and condense them down into a potent mixture of compounds.

WHY USE ESSENTIAL OILS?

There are a slew of reasons why you should use essential oils, but simply put the main reason is because they are good for you. Essential oils work with your body instead of against it. Human beings have co-evolved alongside the plants that are used for their essential oils. Since prehistoric times, humans have been using plants as medicine, and essential oils are the concentrated form of these plants.

The ways in which essential oils benefit us, and how we have used them for generations, is wide and varied. Essential oils can heal wounds; relieve indigestion; kill and inhibit bacteria, viruses, fungi, and parasites; reduce inflammation; detoxify the liver; act as antioxidants by reducing free radicals; relieve pain; soothe irritation; improve mood by reducing stress, anxiety, and depression; help the lymphatic system; repel pests; stimulate our minds; relax our bodies, minds, and muscles; help us sleep; reduce muscle spasms; act as an astringent; deodorize; prevent and reduce the growth of cancer cells; encourage mucus loosening in the lungs; act as a diuretic; reduce blood pressure; affect the nervous system; increase feelings of attraction; increase circulation; stimulate hormone production; and much, much more. Research is still being done on all the benefits of essential oils.

The methodology in which essential oils perform these functions is an important part of why they are beneficial to humans in addition to the plants they derive from. Typical medications are an important part of personal health and many of these medications are derived from plants. Much of the research done on essential oils focuses on their antimicrobial functions against gram-negative (having a thin membrane) and gram-positive (having a thick membrane) bacteria, viruses, fungi, phage, and parasites. One of the reasons that essential oils are so effective against microbes is because they are lipophilic, meaning that they are oil soluble instead of water-soluble. This allows essential oils to interact with cell membranes and affect the behaviors of those cells. Which includes destroying cells that contain viruses or are making us sick.

This ability to interact with cells does not just make essential oils antimicrobial. It also helps them to affect the systems of the human body. Before we had the current scientific methodologies to study and distill essential oils, human beings were using them directly from the plants. Our first ancestors burned herbs and resins as incense. This practice still exists today, but also gave way to creating aromatic oils by steeping herbs, flowers, and resins in oils. The ancient Egyptians and Ayurvedic practitioners in India used these aromatic oils for healing and perfumery. The ancient Egyptians priests even used aromatic oils for mummification and may have had an understanding of distillation. The use of oils for perfumery, religion, and health was passed on to the Ancient Greeks and Romans and even appears multiple times in the Bible. The Arabs brought the final touch of distillation to perfumery and spread this art further around the world. The healing abilities of plants have been researched since that time and that body of knowledge continues to grow today.

Using essential oils gives you the ability to be in control of your health and well-being. They in no way are meant to replace the important relationship you have with your health practitioner, but instead are one of many tools that are necessary to maintain your health. Just as what you eat, where you live, how active you are, and what you do all day affect your health, essential oil use is a choice you make that influences your well-being. Essential oils make for great preventative measures. They give you a place to start on your journey toward a vibrant and healthy lifestyle.

COMMON ESSENTIAL OILS

One of the hardest things about building your essential oil collection is figuring out where to start. Some companies offer such a wide variety of individual essential oils and essential oil blends that sorting through them can easily become overwhelming. The best place to start isn't with the cheapest essential oils, but instead with the oils that have the most versatility and will give you the greatest benefits. You want to build your collection on foundational essential oils that blend well with others and can be used in a wide variety of recipes and protocols. You also want to be sure that the oils you begin with meet your individual well-being needs. Below are details about the ten most prevalent essential oils in this book: lavender, lemon, Roman chamomile, frankincense, orange, melaleuca, bergamot, rosemary, peppermint, and lemongrass. This book contains thirty-five essential oils among the recipes, a collection that would allow you to meet almost all your personal well-being needs. The additional twenty-five essential oils, in order of the number of recipes in which they appear are: geranium, ylang-ylang, clove, sandalwood, lime ginger, basil, cinnamon, vetiver (my personal favorite), black pepper, eucalyptus, cedarwood, myrrh, grapefruit, fennel, oregano, clary sage, marjoram, West Indian bay (a.k.a. bay rum), juniper berry, cypress, thyme, white fir, cardamon, and cilantro. Details about these twenty-five essential oils can be found within the recipes where they occur.

Lavender (*Lavandula angustifolia*): Lavender essential oil is one of the most versatile essential oils available at a reasonable price. This is why it is has also been one of the most popular essential oils since the times of the Ancient Greeks and Romans. Lavender essential oil is distilled from lavender flowers and while the exact composition of the essential oil is dependent on the crop and variations in the distillation process—which is true of all essential oils—the main constituents of lavender essential oil remain the same. The main chemical components of lavender essential oil are the alcohol linalool, which is also referred to as linalol, and the ester linalyl acetate. Much research has been done on the therapeutic properties of linalool, and it has been found to be an anti-inflammatory agent, mood relaxing, and to have a sedative effect on the central nervous system. The other major chemical constituents of lavender essential oil include the monoterpene β-ocimene, the sesquiterpene β-caryophyllene, the phenol terpinen-4-ol, and the oxide 1,8 cineol.

These chemicals, with many other chemical constituents in smaller amounts, work together to create an essential oil that is analgesic, anxiety reducing, antidepressant, anti-inflammatory, antispasmodic, antimicrobial, and sedative. Lavender also has the ability to reduce the perception of pain. Lavender is also one of the safest essential oils for young children. It is very mild and can be used with babies over three months of age. Some people do find that lavender essential oil is not the best essential oil for them. For many lavender cures headache and soothes the skin, but for a few, it causes headaches and irritates the skin. For those who have adverse reactions

IMAGES OF COMMON ESSENTIAL OILS

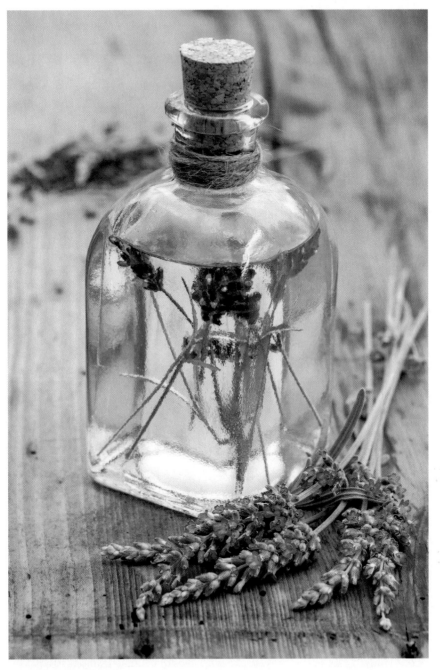

Lavender essential oil

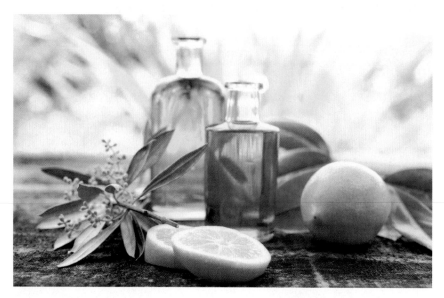

Lemon essential oil

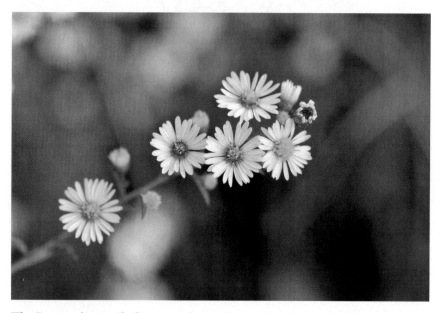

The Roman chamomile flower used to make essential oils

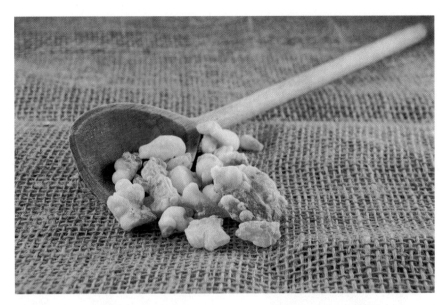

Pictured above is the aromatic resin, Frankincense, which is obtained from the olibanum tree.

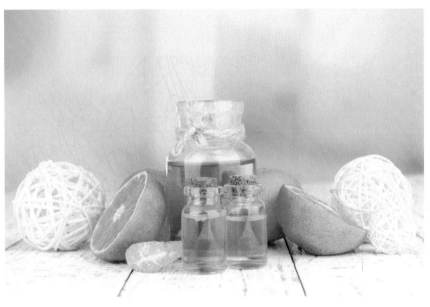

Orange essential oil

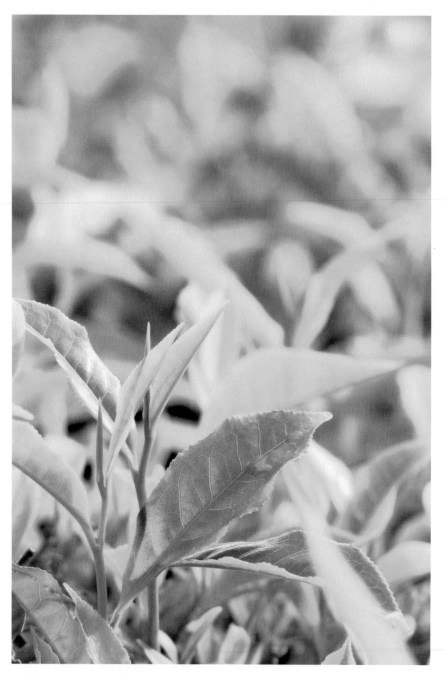

Melaleuca, or tea tree leaves used to make essential oils

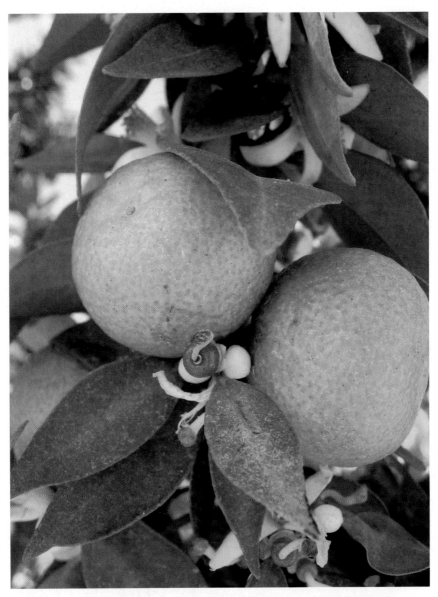

Bergamot oil comes from a citrus tree native to Europe and South East Asia.

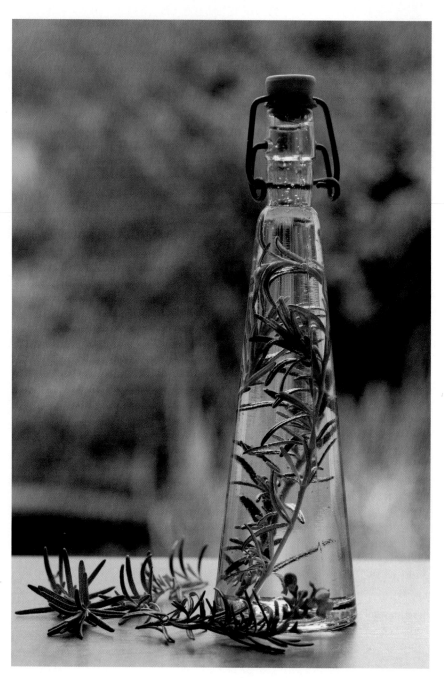

Rosemary essential oil

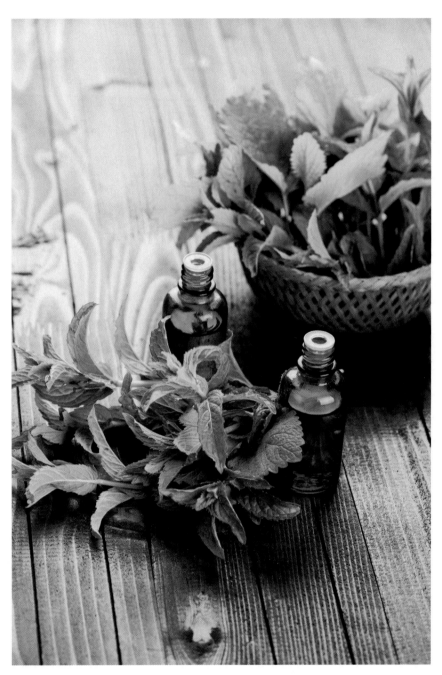

Peppermint essential oil

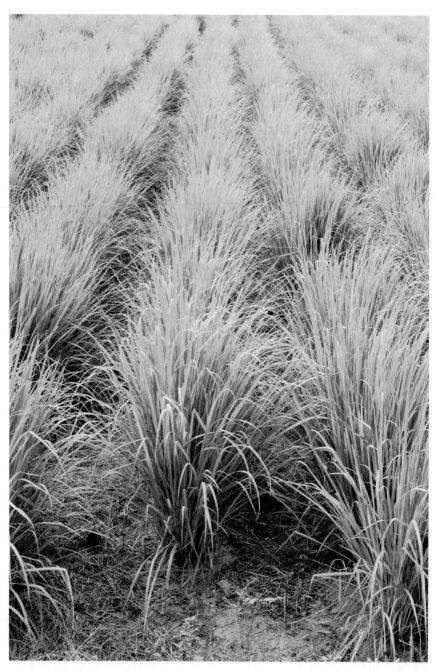

Lemongrass oil comes from the lemongrass plant. Pictured here is a lemongrass field in the northeast of Thailand.

to lavender essential oil, replace it with Roman chamomile or German chamomile for the recipes in this book.

Lemon (*Citrus limon*): Lemons have long been prized for their ability to clean. Lemon essential oil not only cleans surfaces, but also cleanses the body. It does this by stimulating the liver to flush out the essential oil along with toxins that have accumulated within the liver and blood. Lemon essential oil's antioxidant properties also benefit the body. Lemon essential oil cleans household surfaces, the air, and the skin because it is antimicrobial, combating bacteria, viruses, and fungi. Lemon essential oil is also mood enhancing. It invigorates and uplifts the mind, working as an antidepressant and antianxiety agent.

Lemon essential oil is cold-pressed from lemon rinds. This reduces the phototoxicity and photosensitivity that can be associated with citrus oils, but you still want to be careful to rinse off lemon essential oil from your skin before going out in the sun. The main chemical found in lemon essential oil is the monoterpene d-limonene. The other major monoterpenes found in lemon essential oil include α- and β-pinenes, along with α- and γ-terpinenes.

Roman chamomile (*Chamaemelum nobile* a.k.a. *Anthemis nobilis*): Roman chamomile is a perennial plant that is also known as English chamomile, or just plain camomile in England. It looks very similar to the annual plant German chamomile and has many of the same properties (which means if necessary you can substitute German chamomile for Roman chamomile in this book's recipes), but the cone of the Roman chamomile plant is solid while the German chamomile cone is hollow. Like the name suggests, Roman chamomile was used in Ancient Rome and has been popular ever since.

Roman chamomile essential oil is steam distilled from the flowers of the plant. It consists primarily of esters, the most prevalent of which is isobutyl angelate. The properties of Roman chamomile are wide and varied. They include being anti-inflammatory, antispasmodic, antidepressant, sedative, and anti-infectious. Roman chamomile is well known for its digestive and calming benefits. Like lavender, Roman chamomile is gentle and safe for babies as young as three months old.

Frankincense (*Boswellia sacra, Boswellia frereana, Boswellia serrata,* and *Boswellia papyrifera*): There are several therapeutic *Boswellia* species that are used to make essential oils. The essential oil is produced from frankincense olibanum or "tears," which are the harvested resin of boswellia trees. These "tears" are then steam distilled to produce frankincense essential oil. Frankincense essential oil includes phallandrenes, pinenes, thujenes, plus important boswellic acids.

Frankincense has been used medicinally since biblical times and is mentioned frequently in ancient texts. One of the most noted benefits of frankincense essential oil is its cancer preventing properties. Frankincense is also an antioxidant and anti-inflammatory essential oil, which makes it rejuvenating and healing. These properties also benefit the mind, and frankincense is great for combating anxiety and depression. Often frankincense is associated with myrrh, and they have many similar properties. If needed, myrrh can replace frankincense in many recipes.

Orange (*Citrus sinensis*): Known as sweet orange or wild orange, this essential oil is not to be confused with the bitter orange (*Citrus aurantium*). Sweet orange essential oil is extracted from the orange rind, usually through a cold-press method. The essential oil of sweet oranges predominantly contains d-limonene, making it cleansing and incredibly mood lifting. Orange essential oil relieves anxiety and generally encourages feelings of happiness. It also is an antioxidant and antimicrobial essential oil.

Melaleuca (*Melaleuca alternifolia*): Melaleuca essential oil is most commonly known as tea tree oil. Aborigines in Australia and New Zealand have been using the melaleuca tree for generations for its medicinal benefits. This knowledge has been passed on, and melaleuca essential oil is now a well known and commonly used essential oil. It is best known for its antifungal effects, but it also protective against bacterial and viruses. Plus, melaleuca essential oil is an antioxidant and is anti-inflammatory. This makes it a prime essential oil for treating skin infections. Melaleuca essential oil is distilled from the leaves of the melaleuca, or tea, tree. It primarily contains monoterpenes including α- and γ- terpinenes, p-cymene, α- and β-pinenes, along with the phenol terpinene-4-ol.

Bergamot (*Citrus bergamia*): Bergamot is one of the lesser known citrus fruits, but it has an amazing ability to relieve anxiety and stress. Bergamot essential oil has a lower limonene content that other citrus essential oils and has several chemical constituents in common with lavender essential oil including lunalyl acetate, linalool, and geraniol. This is why bergamot is so relaxing, yet energizing. Unlike other citrus essential oils, bergamot is generally solvent extracted instead of cold-pressed. This reduces its phototoxicity to a greater degree than other extraction methods, but bergamot is still considered the most phototoxic essential oil, meaning it should not be left on the skin when going out into the sun. Wash-off bergamot essential oil products are safe and rarely cause problems. Bergamot is a great essential oil to use in the diffuser because of its mood-enhancing benefits.

Rosemary (*Rosmarinus officinalis*): Rosemary essential oil is a strong and powerful essential oil. It is one of the most potent antimicrobial essential oils, with the ability to inhibit viruses, bacteria, fungi, and other microbes. This potency, and its high concentration of 1,8 cineol, means that it is best used by adults. In addition to 1,8 cineol, rosemary essential oil primarily consists of α-and β-pinenes, camphor, β-thujone, verbenone, and borneol. It is analgesic and anti-inflammatory, plus it's great for clearing out congestion from the respiratory system.

Peppermint (*Mentha piperita*): Peppermint is well known as a flavoring agent, but is also used medicinally. Drinking peppermint tea is considered a great way to wake up and ease digestion, but peppermint essential oil is almost thirty times stronger than peppermint tea. Plus, these aren't the only benefits of peppermint. Peppermint is another versatile essential oil with a many, many benefits including—but definitely not limited to!—being analgesic, antimicrobial, antispasmodic, stimulating, and an expectorant. Peppermint is great for headaches, respiration, digestive issues, nausea, and as mentioned earlier, it helps wake you up! The smell of peppermint reminds people of menthol because peppermint essential oil contains a lot of it.

Peppermint is a complex essential oil, containing a wide variety of compounds. In addition to menthol, some of these compounds include menthone, α-and β-pinenes, menthyl acetate, limonene, and 1.8 cineol. The amount of 1.8 cineol in peppermint is much lower than in rosemary, but it is still not recommended for children under the age of six as it can be harsh on their respiratory systems. For younger children, you can stick to peppermint tea or replace the peppermint with lemon or basil essential oils depending on the situation.

Lemongrass (*Cymbopogon flexuosus*): Lemongrass essential oil is not as well known as melaleuca, but it is actually a stronger antifungal agent. Its anti-inflammatory, antimicrobial, analgesic, and vasodilating properties make it great for tissue repair. Plus it is apt at getting rid of smells, cleaning the air and surfaces, improving digestive health, and soothing muscle aches. Lemongrass essential oil is steam distilled from the leaves of the lemongrass plant. This process produces an essential oil that includes the aldehydes geranial and neral, the alcohols geraniol and farnesol, the esters geranyl and linalyl acetates, and the monoterpene myrcene.

METHODS OF USE

There are three main ways to use essential oils: aromatically, topically, and internally. Aromatic use is the most common and well known form of aromatherapy, hence the name. All the essential oils are meant for use aromatically, most are safe and recommended for topical use, and internal use is reserved for fewer of the essential oils available.

Aromatic Use: The fastest way to use essential oils aromatically is to smell them directly from the bottle; however, this is also the least efficient way to use them. Leaving essential oil bottles open causes them to evaporate and does not dissipate the essential oils in an effective manner. You can also pour a couple drops of essential oils into your hand and inhale, but once again while this may be quick, it is not efficient. The best way to use essential oils aromatically is with a diffuser. Essential oil diffusers use water vapor to disperse the essential oils into the air. Quality diffusers do not use heat and therefore do not damage the essential oils during diffusion. Aromatic use of essential oils are ideal for when you want to receive the psychological effects of essential oils because of the close connection between olfactory cells and the brain. Diffuser use is also helpful for cleaning the air and the respiratory system.

Topical Use: Skin is our largest organ, absorbing topical substances directly into our bloodstream. Topical use of essential oils allows the benefits of essential oil use to reach our skin, our organs, and our whole body. When applying essential oils topically for full-body use, the most absorbent point on our bodies is the arch of our foot. To avoid skin sensitivities to essential oils, make sure to dilute the essential oils in a carrier oil. A carrier oil is a stable plant oil such as olive oil, coconut oil, sweet almond oil, avocado oil, jojoba oil, apricot kernel oil, or evening primrose oil. These are just a few of the many carrier oils available at your local grocery or health food store. When diluting essential oils for regular use, you want to find a ratio that works best for your age and skin type. The ratio of essential oil to carrier oil is 1 percent for each drop of essential oil per teaspoon of carrier oil. This means for a 5 percent dilution, which is ideal for typical adult skin, you would use 5 drops of essential oil with a teaspoon of coconut oil. This is not always absolutely exact because drop size is not absolute. Citrus oils tend to release in larger drops than more viscous essential oils, like vetiver and myrrh. Occasionally neat, undiluted use is fine for certain oils, such as lavender on bug bites, but it is important to listen to your body and if your skin starts to feel irritated, be sure to dilute.

Internal Use: Internal use of essential oils is done in several different ways, including suppositories, but the most common of method is oral ingestion. When ingesting essential oils, you MUST be sure than you are using essential oils that are of a high enough quality to ingest and are labeled as such. DO NOT ingest essential oils that say "for external use only" or "do not ingest." Essential oils that are safe for ingestion should have serving information and/ or supplement facts written on the bottle. Dilution is also important when ingesting essential oils. Because essential oils are not water soluble, it is best to dilute them in liquids that contain fats, in honey, in carrier oils, or in capsules combined with carrier oils. Internal use of essential oils is best for flavoring foods and when you are trying to affect your digestive tract.

QUALITY LEVELS

There is no governing body that regulates the quality of essential oils. They are considering supplements and therefore, unregulated by the

FDA. The FDA does prevent essential oil companies from making health claims about the effects of their particular essential oils, even if research backs up those claims, because essential oils are not considered drugs. This has benefits and drawbacks. The first benefit is that essential oils are readily available, and because they are natural products, they cannot be owned or patented by a particular company. Companies can create their own proprietary blends, but single essential oils can be carried by any company. This is great for the educated consumer, but makes it very hard for those new to essential oils to know which products are high quality and which ones are not.

The simplest way to differentiate between essential oil quality is often price, but this is not always true. More expensive essential oils tend to be of higher quality, but some high-quality companies are able to maintain reasonable prices. So if price isn't always a reliable factor what do you do? First, you can look on the bottle for some clues. Food and perfume grade essential oils are not nearly as good as therapeutic grade essential oils, but once again there isn't a governing body that makes that decision. Some companies establish their own markers of quality by sending their oils to third-party testing sites to establish quality. These companies will usually mention this on their packaging or in their informative materials. Another thing to look for when buying essential oils is whether the single essential oils are prediluted. This brings down the price and the quality of the oils. You want to choose oils that are unadulterated, so that you can dilute them to fit your needs.

So where can you buy higher quality essential oils? Well, unfortunately, most high-quality oils need to be bought through a distributor or online. The oils available at local stores tend to be of lower quality due to the price point of the higher quality oils. If you are only using your essential oils for the pleasant aroma and not for the therapeutic benefits, these lower quality oils will suffice. However, when making the recipes in this book, higher quality oils are necessary. There are many companies that carry pure essential oils, and finding a company you trust is important. Companies with good customer service, educational materials, and quality relationships with their suppliers tend to have higher quality essential oils. When a company can tell you about where their essential oils are sourced, what type of growing conditions are required for their oils, who is growing the plants that hold their essential oils, and what the chemical constituents of their essential oils are, that company has an eye on quality.

ESSENTIAL OIL SAFETY

Negative reactions to essential oils are rare, but can occur. The most common, though still rare, negative reactions to essential oils are photosensitivity—an increased sensitivity to sunlight—and allergic contact dermatitis—a rash or irritation of the skin caused by skin contact with an allergen or irritant. Bergamot essential oil has been known to cause photosensitivity and other citrus oils carry the possibility of causing photosensitivity, but reports of them doing so are uncommon. The risk of photosensitivity with citrus oils is also related to how the essential oils are extracted. Steam distillation increases this risk, while cold-press extraction and solvent extraction reduce the phototoxicity of citrus oils. Most citrus essential oils are cold-pressed and bergamot is often solvent extracted, but it is important to check the method of extraction when purchasing and using citrus essential oils. The best way to avoid the risk of photosensitivity from citrus essential oils when using them topically is to dilute them well (less than 0.5 percent dilution) or use them in products that can be washed off after use. Contact dermatitis can be avoided by diluting essential oils appropriately, ceasing to use specific essential oils that cause you irritation, and by rotating which essential oils you use on a regular basis. Certain essential oils—including black pepper, cassia, cinnamon, clove, eucalyptus, ginger, lemongrass, oregano, peppermint, thyme—are considered "hot" oils and can cause a hot or flush feeling on the skin when used undiluted. These oils require additional dilution with carrier oil when used topically. These same oils can cause irritations to the lips, mouth, throat, and stomach if not diluted properly.

Additionally, if you are allergic to the plant from which an essential oil is derived, you may be allergic to the essential oil as well. This allergy may present itself as allergic contact dermatitis or in another manner similar to how your allergy typically presents. If an allergic reaction to an essential oil, due to an existing allergy, is a possibility, there are two options: avoid the essential oil entirely, or perform a spot test on your skin. When testing for allergic contact dermatitis, be sure to heavily dilute the essential oil to a 0.5 percent dilution rate, which equals one drop of essential oil to two teaspoons of carrier oil. If any sensitivity occurs, refrain from using that essential oil. Also, make sure to keep an eye out for sensitivity in the future due to increased exposure.

Topical sensitivities to essential oils are the easiest to spot, but there are other, once again rare, risks when using essential oils on a regular basis. Systemic toxicities can occur over time. Like dermal sensitivities, these systemic toxicities can be avoided by properly diluting essential oils and by rotating which essential oils you use on a regular basis. Proper dilution prevents the body from absorbing potentially toxic levels of essential oils, while rotating your choice of essential oils reduces the chance of essential oil constituents from building up to toxic levels within your body. The systemic risks of essential oils include the risk to the fetus of a pregnant mother using essential oils (fetotoxicity), the risk of tumor formation as a reaction to essential oil use (carcinogenicity), potential liver damage (hepatotoxicity), possible lung damage (pulmonary toxicity), and adverse effects to the nervous system, including the brain (neurotoxicity). The essential oils in this book have not been found to cause these systemic toxicities when used as recommended. Much of the advice about avoiding certain essential oils is theoretical or precautionary, but there are a few essential oils that are available for purchase that should be avoided due to reported instances of systemic toxicity. For example, pennyroyal essential oil has been found to be hepatotoxic and to cause pulmonary toxicity in mice, but this does not mean the same would be true for human use. However, this book errs on the side of caution, and any potential dangers are noted within each recipe. In this same vein, none of the recipes in this book are recommended for pregnant or lactating mothers, or children under the age of six, unless specifically noted.

Keep essential oils out of the reach of children. As well, make sure that your bottles of essential oils have orifice reducers and/or child safety caps, so that if a child manages to get ahold of a bottle of essential oil, the bottle is either unopenable or the flow of essential oil is reduced to the point that the child cannot ingest a toxic amount of the essential oil. While deaths from consumption of essential oils are uncommon, there have been cases of children ingesting entire bottles of essential oils, resulting in hospitalization or even death.

Never put essential oils directly into your eyes!

SUPPLIES TO GET STARTED
WITH ESSENTIAL OILS

When working with essential oils, there are several tools you need to have and safety precautions you need to keep in mind. As mentioned earlier, always keep your essential oils out of the reach of young children. With that in mind a big question is: so where do I keep them? The basic answer is in a cool, dark, and dry place. The ideal place to store your essential oils and essential oil products would be in a still room, but not many houses have those these days. So instead, the refrigerator is a simple alternative, but a cool cupboard also will suffice.

The other important thing to know about when working with essential oils is that you do not want to store essential oils or their products in plastics. Essential oils, especially citrus oils, can react with certain plastics and aluminium and leach unwanted chemicals into your essential oil products. Also, because light can degrade the essential oils, you want to use storage containers that reduce the amount of light that can affect your products. Therefore, the ideal storage containers for essential oil products are blue or amber glass or sturdy metal containers. These types of containers can be found at bottle supply companies, online, or often at local health food stores. For products that are quickly consumed, clear glass containers, such as mason jars, can be used as well.

Along with having the right bottles for storing your products, you want to get the right kinds of tops. When making blends of essential oils, you want to either use 10 mL bottles with roller tops that spread the blend onto the body or 5 or 15 mL glass vials with orifice reducer in the neck of the bottle. Roller bottles are best for blends that have been prediluted, while the vials are appropriate for blends without carrier oils in them. The orifice reducer makes it easier to count the number of drops of essential oil you are using in recipes or for dilution purposes. You can also use glass eye dropper tops for diluted or undiluted blends.

For sprays, you want to get spray bottle tops that fit the size bottle you have stored your product in. One of the important things to remember is that the tubing that brings the liquid up to the spray nozzle is most likely going to be plastic. These plastics are often sturdier than other plastics and less likely to degrade in essential oil products. If you find this is not true, use a different spray nozzle. Also, the tubing may be longer than the bottle you have, so make sure to cut down the tubing to fit your bottle. The same is true for pump tops.

Besides storing your essential oil products, you want to be sure the have the proper materials for making your essential oil recipes. Glass bowls are ideal for preparing many of the recipes in this book. You will want to have a wide variety of bowl sizes available, from small 2-ounce bowls to large mixing bowls. You can use metal spoons, forks, and spatulas—or even electric mixers—for mixing the ingredients together. If you use a wooden spoon or spatula, make sure that it has been properly seasoned. Raw wood will absorb the essential oils out of the recipe you are making.

The final touch for your essential oil products is determining how to label them. Waterproof labels are best for anything you will be using near the bath, shower, or sink, but are not necessary for powder-based items, such as mattress powder. Printable labels are available at office supply stores, while decorative labels that can be handwritten are carried at most craft stores. Beautiful labels are great for gifts and decorating your house, but ultimately making sure that your items are labeled clearly makes life a lot easier.

PART TWO
Essential Oils for Natural Health Care

Seasonal Ailments

FLU BOMB PROTOCOL

The flu, unlike the common cold, usually hits suddenly and seemingly out of the blue. You feel fine, and then within less than an hour, you're achy, feverish, and feel downright miserable. Getting your yearly flu vaccine can help you avoid the flu, but it doesn't always work and we don't always get it in time to prevent catching the latest strain of influenza. Luckily, this flu bomb protocol is there for you the moment you feel that tickle in your throat or ache in your neck that signals an upcoming bout of the flu. One of the other great benefits of this protocol is that it works on the common cold, too! Just make sure you start using it right away. The lower your viral load, the more effective this and any other supportive measure will be. And remember rest, rest, rest, rest, and more rest is the very best way for your body to focus on fighting the flu or any other infection.

There are multiple recipes within this protocol because your body needs multiple means of support when it is fighting off the flu. The recipes are listed with ingredients, preparation, and administration first, but use them all for the entire protocol. Benefits for the entire protocol and additional notes are given after the recipes.

ANTIMICROBIAL WATER
Ingredients:

16 ounces of water

1 teaspoon honey

1 drop lemon essential oil

1 drop cinnamon essential oil

1 drop lemongrass essential oil

Preparation:
1. In a pint glass, combine 1 teaspoon of honey and 1 drop each of lemon, cinnamon, and lemongrass essential oils.
2. Add 16 ounces of water.

Administration:
1. Drink the entire contents of the pint glass.

FLU FIGHTING GARGLE
Ingredients:

1 ounce water
1 drop clove essential oil
1 drop rosemary essential oil
1 drop oregano essential oil
1 drop lemon essential oil
1 drop melaleuca essential oil
1 drop cinnamon essential oil

Preparation:
1. In a 2-ounce glass, add one drop each of clove, rosemary, oregano, lemon, melaleuca, and cinnamon essential oils to 1 ounce of water.

Administration:
1. Pour the Flu Fighting Gargle into your mouth toward your throat.
2. Gargle for 1–2 minutes.
3. Spit.

FLU FIGHTING NECK AND CHEST RUB
Ingredients:

2 teaspoons sweet almond oil (or other carrier oil)
3 drops cypress essential oil
2 drops black pepper essential oil
2 drops melaleuca essential oil
1 drop basil essential oil

Preparation and administration:
1. Take caps off essential oil bottles.
2. Pour 2 teaspoons sweet almond oil into the palm of your hand.
3. Add 3 drops cypress, 2 drops black pepper, 2 drops melaleuca, and 1 drop basil essential oils.
4. Rub your hands together, then rub your shoulders, neck, and chest with the Flu Fighting Neck and Chest Rub.

5. Replace the caps on the essential oil bottles.
6. Inhale the aroma of the rub.

FLU FIGHTING FOOT RUB
Ingredients:
1 tablespoon extra-virgin olive oil

1 medium-large garlic clove, crushed

1 drop oregano essential oil

Preparation:
1. Use a garlic press to crush 1 medium-large garlic clove.
2. Scrape crushed garlic into a small glass bowl.
3. Add 1 tablespoon extra-virgin olive oil.
4. Mix in 1 drop oregano essential oil.

Administration:
1. Scoop a portion of the Flu Fighting Foot Rub into your hand.
2. Rub onto the bottoms of your feet.
3. Rub between your toes to stimulate the reflexology points for your lymphatic system.
4. Focus on the outer balls of your feet to activate the reflexology points for your lungs.
5. Scoop the rest of the Flu Fighting Foot Rub into your hand and massage your entire foot.
6. Put on clean socks.

SOUP ENHANCER
Ingredients:
2 cups chicken noodle soup

1 tablespoon extra-virgin olive oil

1 medium-large clove garlic, minced

2 drops lemon essential oil

2 drops black pepper essential oil

Preparation:
1. Heat 2 cups of your favorite chicken noodle soup and 1 medium-large minced clove of garlic on the stove.

2. While the soup is heating, in a small glass bowl, combine 1 tablespoon extra-virgin olive oil and 2 drops each of lemon and black pepper essential oils.
3. Once soup is evenly heated, remove from the stove and pour into a bowl (not plastic).
4. Allow to cool to a consumable temperature, then add oil mixture. Stir.

Administration:
1. Snuggle up and eat your soup as you inhale the steam it produces.

Benefits:
Cinnamon and lemongrass essential oils are highly antimicrobial against viruses, bacteria, fungi, and protozoans.

Clove, oregano, rosemary, lemon, basil, and melaleuca essential oils have a wide range of antimicrobial effects, both killing and inhibiting a variety of bacteria, viruses, and fungi.

Cypress and basil essential oils are stimulating to the respiratory and cardiovascular systems.

Garlic contains the antimicrobial agent allicin, which can be absorbed into the bloodstream through the pores in the feet.

Olive oil's antioxidant rich phenolic compounds, hydroxytyrosol and oleuropein, contribute to the body's ability to fight off infections.

Chicken noodle soup is one of the most comforting foods to eat when we are sick. That comfort improves how we feel while we are battling illness. Additionally, the steam from the soup relieves congestion and soothes the throat.

Lemon essential oil stimulates the liver, which improves overall health.

Black pepper is the most commonly used spice, not just due to its taste, but also because of its medicinal properties. Black pepper essential oil contains pet ether, a highly antioxidant substance, with health benefits ranging from anticancer to immunological support.

Notes and Tips:
Diffuse the Winter Diffuser Blend (page 23) for additional flu fighting benefits.

CAUTION: Use lip balm before drinking the Antimicrobial Water to reduce irritation to the lips.

WINTER DIFFUSER BLEND

Winter is known as cold and flu season, but it's not just colds or the flu that get us sick in the winter. While viruses thrive in cold, dry weather, bacteria love to move from person to person when we are confined in closer quarters. Throw in some secondary bacterial infections and you've got yourself a cauldron of illnesses. Instead of wrangling with being sick, turn on your diffuser and enjoy the festive aroma.

Ingredients:
½ cup water
4 drops cinnamon essential oil
3 drops clove essential oil
2 drops orange essential oil
2 drops bergamot essential oil
1 drop rosemary essential oil

Preparation and Administration:
1. Pour ½ cup of water into the water container of your diffuser (or the amount needed by your particular brand of diffuser).
2. Add 4 drops cinnamon, 3 drops clove, 2 drops orange, 2 drops bergamot, and 1 drop rosemary essential oil to the water in the diffuser.
3. Place your diffuser in a central location in the room.
4. Turn on your diffuser and allow the room to fill aroma of the Winter Diffuser Blend.

Benefits:
Cinnamon and clove are two of the most highly antimicrobial essential oils. With their ability to kill a wide range of infection-causing microbes, it's no surprise they are winter favorites.

Citrus oils, like orange and bergamot, are excellent at cleansing the air. The aroma of oranges pairs well with cinnamon and clove.

Rosemary essential oil improves respiratory function, which is helpful when seasonal threats are high.

Notes and Tips:
1. If your diffuser is one that is safe to be left on when you are not home, try running your diffuser when you leave the house to cleanse the air while you are gone.
2. The Winter Diffuser Blend is a great way to make your house smell festive when entertaining company—but not their germs—during the holidays.

SORE THROAT GARGLE

Causes of sore throats vary from overuse, abrasion, allergies, and most commonly, infection. When caused by an infection, a sore throat is often the first sign that more severe symptoms are on the way. A sore throat is irritating, but also makes swallowing and talking difficult and painful. This sore throat gargle both soothes the pain of a sore throat and supports healing of the irritation or infection.

Ingredients:
2 teaspoons raw honey (preferably local)
1 ounce water
1 drop clove essential oil
1 drop cinnamon essential oil

Preparation:
1. Mix the two teaspoons of raw honey and the ounce of water into a small saucepan and warm over low heat just enough to melt the honey.
2. Pour the honey/water mixture into a 2-ounce glass.
3. Add 1 drop each of clove and cinnamon essential oils.

Administration:
1. Pour the Sore Throat Gargle into your mouth toward your throat.
2. Gargle for 1–2 minutes.
3. Spit.

Benefits:
Honey has been used for thousands of years for wound treatments, and those properties that make it ideal for external wounds—specifically the antibacterial and anti-inflammatory properties—also, make it ideal for supporting the healing of a sore throat.

The role of local raw honey in relieving the symptoms of seasonal allergies is beginning to be studied with some results showing a decrease in rhinitis symptoms. If the sore throat is caused by postnasal drip, using local raw honey gives this recipe additional benefits.

The clove bud essential oil in this recipe is essential for the analgesic, or numbing, properties of this gargle. The clove bud essential oil numbs the throat, therefore, relieving the pain felt while swallowing. The anti-inflammatory properties further soothe the throat by reducing any swelling. Additionally, clove bud essential oil has antibacterial, antiviral, and antifungal properties.

Cinnamon bark essential oil has been found to effectively inhibit the growth of candida and both gram-positive and gram-negative bacteria.

Notes and Tips:

Applying a lip balm before using this gargle reduces the risk that the numbing effects of the clove bud essential oil or the "hot" effect of the cinnamon bark essential oil will affect your lips.

LARYNGITIS GARGLE

Losing your voice is more than just a minor side effect of an inflamed voice box—it affects your ability to communicate with the world around you. Attempting to speak softly just irritates your voice box more, making your laryngitis worse. Laryngitis has many potential causes, from too much shouting at a sporting event to infection, but no matter the cause, the result is painful and debilitating. This gargle is not intended to treat medical causes of your laryngitis, but instead to give you relief from the pain and soothe your vocal chords enough for you to call the doctor. If you know you are recovering from overuse of your voice, then this will accelerate that recovery.

Ingredients:

1 tablespoon virgin coconut oil
1 drop lavender essential oil
1 drop Roman chamomile essential oil
1 drop frankincense essential oil

Preparation:

1. Warm 1 tablespoon coconut oil just enough to melt it. This can be done in a glass container in the microwave for 10 seconds at a time until melted or on the stove on low heat in under a minute.
2. Pour the melted coconut oil into a 1-ounce glass.
3. Add 1 drop each of lavender, Roman chamomile, and frankincense essential oils.

Administration:

1. Pour the Laryngitis Gargle into your mouth toward your throat.
2. Gargle for 1–2 minutes.
3. Spit.

Benefits:

Coconut oil has a mild analgesic and anti-inflammatory effects, making it an ideal carrier oil for this gargle.

Lavender essential oil is soothing for any type of pain and has been specifically tested on throat pain and been found to reduce the need for additional analgesics.

Chamomile is both anti-inflammatory and antispasmodic. It is ideal for soothing inflammation of mucous membranes. The antibacterial properties are an added benefit if your laryngitis is the result of a bacterial infection.

Frankincense essential oil is also prized for its anti-inflammatory properties. Its ability to aid in respiratory health increases the benefits of this laryngitis gargle.

Notes and Tips:

This gargle is safe to swallow after use, but this will not significantly increase its effectiveness.

HEAD COLD TEA

Sometimes when you get sick, it feels like your nasal cavities are fighting the virus all by themselves. The rest of your body feels fine, but your head feels ready to explode. This head cold tea will help clear your nasal cavities and support your immune system.

Ingredients:
1 ½ cups water
2 green onions
1 drop ginger essential oil

Preparation:
1. Heat water in a pan on high heat until it boils.
2. Reduce heat and add 2 green onions. Let onions simmer, covered, for five minutes.
3. Strain onion broth into a ceramic mug and let cool.
4. When the broth is close to a drinkable temperature, but still steaming, add one drop of ginger essential oil and stir with a metal spoon.

Administration:
1. Inhale the steam from the mug for approximately one minute.
2. Drink the green onion and ginger essential oil mixture when it is cool enough to drink, but still warm.

Benefits:
Green onion and ginger root "tea" is a common folk remedy for colds. This recipe brings the concentrated benefits of ginger essential oil to the traditional recipe.

Ginger essential oil has both antiviral properties and immune supporting properties. This combination makes it ideal for supporting the body while it fights off the common cold.

Notes and Tips:
Ginger essential oil is considered a "hot" oil, which means it can cause skin irritation if not diluted properly. One drop of ginger essential oil is all that is needed for this tea. Adding more essential oil will make it uncomfortable to drink, so be cautious.

Make sure to add the ginger essential oil last because essential oils are damaged by high heat and adding the ginger essential oil to boiling water would reduce its potency. This mixture may be consumed multiple times for continued support. About every two hours is ideal, but every person is different, as is every ailment, so listen to your body to know if you need to drink this tea more or less often.

CHEST CONGESTION PROTOCOL

Congestion affects the entire respiratory system from the nose to the lungs, even affecting the ears at times. Mucus forms to reduce irritation and trap infections, but then the body must rid itself of the mucus. Using essential oils to fight the infections themselves and to expel the mucus from the body frees up the respiratory system to do what it does best: breathe.

BREATH OF FRESH AIR BLEND
Ingredients:
24 drops lemon essential oil

16 drops peppermint essential oil

16 drops eucalyptus essential oil

12 drops juniper berry essential oil

12 drops cardamom essential oil

Preparation:
1. In a 5 mL amber glass vial, combine 24 drops lemon, 16 drops peppermint, 16 drops eucalyptus, 12 drops juniper berry, and 12 drops cardamom essential oils.
2. Insert orifice reducer and apply cap.
3. Shake well.

SHOWER STEAMERS
Ingredients:
2 cups baking soda

1 cup citric acid

2 tablespoons water

20 drops Breath of Fresh Air Blend, divided

Preparation:
1. In a large bowl, combine 2 cups baking soda and 1 cup citric acid. Stir well with a large metal spoon.
2. In a glass vial or small glass bowl, combine 2 tablespoons water and 10 drops Breath of Fresh Air Blend.
3. Add liquid mixture to the bowl of dry ingredients a few drops at a time, stirring between each addition of liquid.

4. Once all the liquid has been added and the mixture is even, use the spoon to scoop the mixture into ten silicone cupcake molds.
5. Fill each cupcake mold and use the spoon to press the mixture into the mold as you are filling it.
6. Once all the molds are filled, apply more pressure to each shower steamer.
7. Allow to dry in the open air for 24 hours.
8. Once completely dry, remove each shower steamer from its mold.
9. Apply one drop of the Breath of Fresh Air Blend to each shower steamer before storing it in an airtight glass container.

Administration:
1. Remove one shower steamer disk from the glass storage container.
2. Turn on shower and let it get warm/hot.
3. Place shower steamer in the path of the water flow—on the side of the shower, in your hand, or on the floor of the shower.
4. Get into the shower and inhale the aromatherapy steam released by the shower steamer.

VAPOR RUB
Ingredients:
3 tablespoons coconut oil
1 tablespoon cocoa butter
1 tablespoon beeswax
50 drops Breath of Fresh Air Blend

Preparation:
1. Create a double boiler by putting a small glass bowl into a saucepan 1 inch full of water.
2. Over medium heat, bring the water to a simmer.
3. Melt 3 tablespoons coconut oil and 1 tablespoon cocoa butter in the glass bowl.
4. Once melted, add 1 tablespoon beeswax and heat until melted.
5. Remove glass from heat and allow mixture to cool for 4–6 minutes (making sure it's still liquified).
6. Add 50 drops of Breath of Fresh Air Blend and stir.

7. Pour Vapor Rub into a metal or glass container and allow to cool.
8. Cap with an airtight lid.

Administration:
1. Rub vapor rub on chest.
2. Rub vapor rub on the bottoms of feet and apply socks.

Benefits:
Lemon and juniper essential oils cleanse the respiratory system.

Peppermint, cardamom, and eucalyptus essential oils are commonly used for respiratory health. Eucalyptus is an expectorant, which help to loosen mucus. Peppermint and cardamom stimulate the lungs and bronchial tubes. They are also effective against respiratory tract infections.

Notes and Tips:
Ten drops of the Breath of Fresh Air Blend can also be used in a diffuser for the same benefits without the shower.

The amounts listed for the Breath of Fresh Air Blend are enough for four sets of shower steamers, eight uses in the diffuser, or one vapor rub (plus a set of shower steamers and a use in the diffuser).

Empty essential oil vials are perfect for making and storing blends. Use a vial that previously held one of the essential oils in the blend so that you don't have to wash it out or worry about contaminating your blend.

SINUSITIS RINSE

Sinusitis, also known as a sinus infection or rhinosinusitis, can be a chronic or acute problem that causes quite the headache—along with plenty of other aches and irritating symptoms! Viral, bacterial, or fungal infections, along with allergies and blocked nasal passages, are all potential causes of inflamed sinuses that can result in congestion, throbbing headaches, jaw and tooth pain, ear aches, sore throats, facial tenderness, coughing, and fatigue. This sinusitis rinse irrigates the sinuses and clears out the mucus, along with the infections, that block the sinuses and cause much of the pressure associated with sinusitis. The essential oils included in this rinse reduce the inflammation of the nasal passages and the respiratory system, which mitigate the painful symptoms experienced by those with sinusitis.

Ingredients:
1 cup warm distilled or sterile water
½ teaspoon salt
2 drops eucalyptus essential oil
2 drops rosemary essential oil
2 drops geranium essential oil
1 drop melaleuca essential oil

Preparation:
1. Add 1 cup of warm water to a neti pot, or other nasal irrigation device.
2. Stir 1 tablespoon of salt into the warm water.
3. Add 2 drops each of eucalyptus and rosemary essential oils.
4. Add 1 drop of melaleuca essential oil.
5. Put cap on neti pot, cover spout, and shake to mix salt, water, and essential oils thoroughly.

Administration:
1. Over a sink, shower drain, or glass bowl, tilt your head to the side at an angle of approximately 45 degrees.
2. Place the spout of the neti pot into your nostril and pour the contents of the neti pot into your nostril so the rinse flows through your nasal cavity and out your other nostril. (If the contents flow down into your throat, spit the rinse and any mucus out through your mouth.)
3. Once the entire contents of the neti pot have been emptied into your nostril, remove the neti pot, press your finger against your nostril to create a vacuum, and blow any remaining mucus out of your other nostril.
4. Make another batch of the Sinusitis Rinse and repeat through the other nostril.

Benefits:
Eucalyptus and rosemary essential oils are commonly used for respiratory health, and the sinuses are an important part of the respiratory system. They are both expectorants, which help to loosen mucus.

Eucalyptus, rosemary, and melaleuca essential oils are all antiviral and antibacterial.

Geranium, rosemary, and eucalyptus essential oils' anti-inflammatory properties reduce the pressure associated with sinusitis.

Additionally, geranium, rosemary, and melaleuca essential oils are strong antifungal agents.

Notes and Tips:

You can sterilize your water simply by boiling it and letting it cool to a lukewarm temperature before adding it to your neti pot.

When irrigating your sinuses, you want to be sure to have a place for the water to run out of your nose (along with the mucus). Using your neti pot while at the end of a warm shower allows the steam from your shower to loosen the mucus in advance. Plus, the water and mucus will run down the drain along with the rest of the shower water.

Irrigating your sinuses can be uncomfortable for some people, and adding strong essential oils can add an extra sting to the feeling. If the irrigation process feels too harsh, reduce the number of drops of eucalyptus, rosemary, and geranium to one drop each. You can also add one drop of lavender and/or Roman chamomile essential oil to soothe the nasal passageways.

Since chronic sinusitis can be caused by environmental fungi, diffusing geranium and rosemary essential oils in the home can prevent recurring fungal infections.

This entire recipe—minus the salt—can also be used as a diffuser blend. You will just need to adjust the amount of water to work with your particular diffuser.

For sinusitis associated with hay fever, try the Hay Fever Relief Protocol (page 32).

Make sure to thoroughly rinse your neti pot and let it completely air dry before storing it.

HAY FEVER RELIEF PROTOCOL

Hay fever season has been getting progressively worse each year. For the millions of sufferers of allergic rhinitis, this means stuffed-up noses plus sore throats and coughs from postnasal drips. Staying inside all spring, summer, and fall—with completely filtered air—isn't exactly feasible. Complement your other hay fever relief techniques with the Hay Fever Relief Protocol.

INGESTIBLE HAY FEVER RELIEF
Ingredients:

1 tablespoon local wild raw honey

1 drop peppermint essential oil

1 drop lemon essential oil

1 drop lavender essential oil

Preparation and Administration:
1. Pour 1 tablespoon local wild raw honey into a large metal spoon.
2. Add 1 drop each of peppermint, lemon, and lavender essential oils.
3. Swallow mixture.

HAY FEVER RELIEF DIFFUSER BLEND
Ingredients:

water

4 drops lavender essential oil

4 drops lemon essential oil

4 drops peppermint essential oil

Preparation and administration:
1. Fill your diffuser with water to the fill line.
2. Add 4 drops each of lavender, lemon, and peppermint essential oils.
3. Turn on diffuser.
4. Inhale vapors released by the diffuser.

Benefits:
Consuming local honey can reduce the allergic reactions to local pollen.

Lemon cleanses the air and body.

Peppermint opens your airways and reduces the effects of allergic rhinitis.

Lavender is anti-inflammatory and soothes irritated nasal passageways.

Notes and Tips:
This protocol is intended for children and adults over the age of six years old. For children between six months and six years, simply omit the

peppermint essential oil in the Hay Fever Relief Diffuser Blend and do not administer the Ingestible Hay Fever Relief. Instead, blend one drop each of lavender and lemon essential oils in a teaspoon of carrier oil and rub on the child's chest.

Aches and Pains

PAIN RELIEVING BATH SALTS

Balneotherapy, the therapeutic use of mineral salts in warm/hot water, has been used for thousands of years and only had a brief period of time in the last century when it was not used for pain treatment in American medicine. As more scientific research is being done on its benefits, this form of pain management is becoming increasingly popular in the Western medical and holistic communities. The hot water used in balneotherapy relaxes the muscles and reduces the perception of pain. The mineral salts are absorbed by the skin and further soothe muscles and relieve pain. Balneotherapy has been found to be effective in the soothing of osteoarthritis, rheumatoid arthritis, lower back pain, and fibromyalgia.

Ingredients:
¾ cup mineral salts
4 drops peppermint essential oil
4 drops lavender essential oil
3 drops rosemary essential oil
2 drops black pepper essential oil
2 drops frankincense essential oil
2 drops lemongrass essential oil
1 drop myrrh essential oil

Preparation:
1. Pour ¾ cup of mineral salts into a large glass bowl.
2. Drop by drop, mix in 4 drops peppermint, 4 drops lavender, 3 drops rosemary, 2 drops black pepper, 2 drops frankincense, 2 drops lemongrass, and 1 drop myrrh essential oils.
3. Mix thoroughly.
4. Divide between two 4-ounce mason jars.
5. Apply and tighten lids.
6. Label jars.

Administration:
1. Begin drawing a bath with water that is as hot as you can tolerate.
2. Add 2–3 tablespoons of Pain Relieving Bath Salts to your bath when it is about halfway full.
3. Get in the bath and stir the bathwater with your hands so that the salts dissolve as the tub fills to your desired depth.
4. Lay back and soak your body in the salt bathwater. Try to get as much of your body under the surface of the water as possible.
5. Top off the hot water as needed.

Benefits:
Balneotherapy, along with frankincense, Roman chamomile, myrrh, lemongrass, and lavender essential oils reduce the inflammation associated with arthritic conditions.

People with fibromyalgia report fewer tender points after balneotherapy and the use of lavender essential oil.

Inhalation of lavender and rosemary essential oils reduces the perception of pain.

Lemongrass and lavender essential oils are both analgesic essential oils.

A combination of rosemary, peppermint, black pepper, and lavender reduces neck pain.

Notes and Tips:
Balneotherapy works best with water above 68°F (20°C).

Stretching your muscles during your bath will also help to release tension and increase the benefits of your bath.

If stored in a cool, dark place, these bath salts can last for two years or more. Just be sure to keep the lid on tightly. The more often you open the jar, the less effective the bath salts will become due to evaporation of the essential oils.

HEADACHE TEMPLE RUB

Headaches come in a range of intensities, none of them pleasant. Often they start out mild and intensify with time. Use the Headache Temple Rub on the onset of a headache to stop it in its tracks. The head massage increases the absorption of the essential oils and supports their headache-relieving properties. Plus, giving yourself a head massage forces you to stop and decompress.

Ingredients:

1 teaspoon sweet almond oil (or other carrier oil)
1 drop peppermint essential oil
1 drop lavender essential oil
1 drop frankincense essential oil

Preparation:

1. Pour 1 teaspoon sweet almond oil into the palm of your nondominant hand.
2. Add one drop each of peppermint, lavender, and frankincense essential oils.
3. Use the fingers of your dominant hand to mix the oils together and to evenly distribute the mixture onto the fingertips of both hands (excluding the thumbs).

Administration:

1. Begin by placing the fingertips of both hands (excluding the thumbs) at the top-center of the forehead—along the hairline—with the pinkies of each hand touching.
2. Apply steady pressure to your forehead as you take five long, deep breaths through your nose, inhaling the aroma of the essential oils.
3. Reduce the amount of pressure you are applying, but maintain a firm touch.
4. Slowly separate your hands as you sweep your fingertips downward along your hairline toward your temples. Stop when your middle finger is even with the corner of your eyes, but be sure to keep your fingers away from your eyes.
5. Apply firm pressure to your temples and take another five long, deep breaths through your nose.
6. Lift your pinky and ring fingers and use your middle and index fingers to massage your temples in a circular motion.
7. Place your finger at the center of your forehead with your nails touching and your fingers stacked vertically so that your index fingers

are closest to your hairline and your pinkies are closest to your eyebrows.

8. Gently stroke outward in a horizontal motion toward the sides of your head.
9. Repeat steps 7–8 five times.
10. Repeat steps 1–6.
11. Use your thumbs to apply pressure to the spaces between the very top of your spine and the base of your skull. These areas about even with the bottoms of your ears.
12. Use your fingertips to gently stroke the back of your neck. If this area is sensitive, keep the pressure very light.

Benefits:

Peppermint essential oil affects headaches through multiple mechanisms. First, it has a cooling effect on the skin, which changes your perception of the headache. Second, it relaxes your muscles, which reduces the tension around your temples, forehead, and scalp. Finally, the kicker here, peppermint essential oil has an analgesic effect, which reduces the pain you feel, hence reducing the headache.

Lavender essential oil is traditionally used to relieve headaches and scientific research has shown that it works well in reducing headache intensity. Lavender changes our perception of pain, reduces stress, and lowers blood pressure. All of these benefits factor into its ability to alleviate your headache.

Frankincense has been used for millennia to treat headaches. The boswellic acid found in frankincense essential oil works as an anti-inflammatory agent. Consistent use of frankincense essential oil can also prevent future headaches.

Massage and deep breathing in and of themselves reduce tension and soothe headache, but they also increase the effectiveness of the essential oils by driving the oils deeper into the skin and muscles and by allowing the essential oils to reach the brain through the olfactory system.

Notes and Tips:

Caution: Peppermint essential oil is not recommended for children under the age of six. However, this recipe and technique can be used with younger children if the peppermint essential is not included and the sweet almond oil is doubled to two teaspoons.

Peppermint essential oil can be irritating to the eyes, so be careful not to get it on or in your eyes. If the headache relieving blend gets in your eyes, DO NOT flush with water. Instead, wash your hands and use the sweet almond oil to flush out the essential oils.

For people with sensitivities to lavender, the lavender essential oil can be omitted or replaced by Roman chamomile essential oil.

MENSTRUAL RELIEF MASSAGE BLEND

Menstrual cramping and pain can range from mild to crippling. Painful menstruation is referred to as dysmenorrhea, which can negatively affect the daily lives of women around the world. Essential oils and massage have long been used to combat the pain and cramping associated with dysmenorrhea. The Menstrual Relief Massage Blend soothes menstrual pain, reduces menstrual cramping, and even helps with potential mood effects of the menstrual cycle.

Ingredients:
1 tablespoon virgin coconut oil
3 drops geranium essential oil
3 drops ginger essential oil
3 drops lavender essential oil
2 drops clary sage essential oil
2 drops fennel essential oil
2 drops marjoram essential oil
1 drop cinnamon essential oil
1 drop clove essential oil

Preparation:
1. Put 1 tablespoon virgin coconut oil into a small glass, ceramic, or metal container.
2. Add 3 drops each of geranium, ginger, and lavender essential oils.
3. Add 2 drops each of clary sage, fennel, and marjoram essential oils.

4. Add 1 drop each cinnamon and clove essential oils.
5. Mix well with a metal spoon or fork.

Administration:
1. Pour ⅓-½ the Menstrual Relief Massage Blend into your hand.
2. Massage into your pelvic region.
3. Pour another ⅓-½ the Menstrual Relief Massage Blend into your hand.
4. Massage into your lower back.
5. Use the rest of the Menstrual Relief Massage Blend to focus on any areas with particular cramping or pain.

Benefits:
Clove, marjoram, and lavender essential oils are analgesics and reduce the sensation of pain. Lavender also plays a psychological role in the perception of pain by reducing anxiety about pain and by affecting the way the brain acknowledges feelings of pain.
Clary sage and geranium are hormone-balancing essential oils. They reduce pain and mood imbalances that result from menstruation.
Ginger and cinnamon are warming, anti-inflammatory essential oils.
Fennel essential oil reduces overconstriction of the uterus, which reduces the cramping and pain associated with menstruation.
Virgin coconut oil has analgesic and anti-inflammatory properties.

Notes and Tips:
The essential oil portion of the Menstrual Relief Massage Blend can be made in a larger batch and stored in a blue or amber vial. This blend can last for over a year and be used as needed. When using this blend from a larger batch, shake well and mix 15 drops of the Menstrual Relief Massage Blend with 1 tablespoon virgin coconut oil.

ARTHRITIS JOINT RUB

Arthritis is a painful condition that comes in multiple forms, most prevalently osteoarthritis and rheumatoid arthritis. These two forms of arthritis have different causes: wear and tear causes osteoarthritis, while rheumatoid arthritis is an autoimmune disease. However, both forms of arthritis cause joint pain and inflammation. Massage can reduce the severity of both types of arthritis. Adding essential oils to massage improves the anti-inflammatory and pain management aspects of massage.

Ingredients:
1 teaspoon sesame oil
1 drop frankincense essential oil
1 drop ginger essential oil
1 drop juniper berry essential oil
1 drop myrrh essential oil
1 drop Roman chamomile essential oil

Preparation and Administration:
1. Remove the caps from the oil bottles.
2. In the palm of your hand, pour 1 teaspoon sesame oil.
3. Add one drop each of frankincense, ginger, juniper berry, myrrh, and Roman chamomile essential oils.
4. Massage the Arthritis Joint Rub into any joints affected by arthritis.
5. Recap the oil bottles.

Benefits:
Sesame oil works as an analgesic and has been found to relieve the inflammation associated with arthritis.

Roman chamomile is anti-inflammatory and relieves rheumatic pain.

Frankincense supports the maintenance of cartilage, therefore slowing down the progression of osteoarthritis.

Myrrh is traditionally used in India, East Africa, and Saudi Arabia to treat rheumatoid arthritis due to its anti-inflammatory properties.

Juniper and ginger essential oils are antinociceptive, inhibiting the sensation of pain. Like the other essential oils in this recipe, they also have anti-inflammatory properties.

Notes and Tips:
If your arthritis pain prevents you from massaging yourself, have someone you trust administer the Arthritis Joint Rub.

The Pain-Relieving Bath Salts (page 35) can also be helpful for arthritic pain.

This rub can be made in a larger batch and used as needed. Triple the recipe and store in a 10 mL roller bottle. Make sure to keep the roller bottle in a cool, dry, and dark place.

CUT, SCRAPE, AND BURN SALVE

Even adults manage to get cuts, scrapes, and burns in our daily lives. Often we just wash them off and go on our way, but properly caring for these minor wounds can prevent infection and make us feel better. There's no need to just grin and bear it when this cut, scrape, and burn salve will soothe the pain, reduce inflammation, help your body heal, and prevent infection.

Ingredients:
⅓ cup raw honey
1 tablespoon virgin coconut oil
2 tablespoons aloe vera gel
30 drops lavender essential oil
20 drops melaleuca essential oil
15 drops frankincense essential oil
10 drops Roman chamomile essential oil
5 drops clove essential oil

Preparation:
1. In a small glass bowl, pour ⅓ cup raw honey.
2. Add 1 tablespoon virgin coconut oil.
3. Stir in 2 tablespoons aloe vera gel.
4. Use a hand mixer to whisk together the honey, coconut, and aloe vera gel.
5. Stir in 30 drops lavender, 20 drops melaleuca, 15 drops frankincense, 10 drops Roman chamomile, and 5 drops clove.
6. Scoop Cut, Scrape, and Burn Salve into a 4-ounce glass mason jar and store in the refrigerator.

Administration:
1. After cleansing your cut, scrape, or burn, apply a small amount of the Cut, Scrape, and Burn Salve to your wound.
2. Cover with a bandage.

Benefits:

Honey has been used to treat wounds since Ancient Egypt due to its antibacterial properties.

Coconut oil is antimicrobial, anti-inflammatory, and can help relieve mild pain.

Lavender and clove essential oils reduce pain due to their analgesic properties.

Clove and melaleuca essential oils are cleansing and prevent infection. Clove is one of the most antimicrobial essential oils available.

Frankincense and Roman chamomile essential soothe wounds and help them heal due to their antioxidant and anti-inflammatory properties.

Notes and Tips:

This salve is intended for those over the age of two. For younger children, babies over six months, and those who hate to be sticky use the Owie Calming Spray (page 94).

Be careful not to get any water in the salve as this will cause the honey and coconut oils to become rancid.

This salve can be stored in the fridge for up to a year.

STING AND BITE COMPRESS

Bee, wasps, and hornet stings hurt a lot, while bug bites from just about any insect or spider can be terribly itchy and even painful. The more we touch or scratch these bug-related injuries, the worse they get. They start to itch and hurt more and can even become infected. It is important to clean the sting or bite, along with soothing the area. The Sting and Bite Compress cleans WHILE reducing pain and itching.

Ingredients:

¼ cup apple cider vinegar, cold

5 drops lavender essential oil, plus 1 additional drop lavender essential oil per bite/sting

5 drops Roman chamomile essential oil

5 drops Rosemary essential oil (for adults only)

ice

Compress Preparation:
1. Pour ¼ cup cold apple cider vinegar into a glass bowl.
2. Add 5 drops each lavender, Roman chamomile, and rosemary essential oil.
3. Soak a small washcloth in the mixture.

Application:
1. Take washcloth out of compress mixture and wring it out slightly so that it remains wet, but not dripping.
2. Fill the washcloth with ice.
3. Apply ice-filled washcloth to sting or bite area and hold there until the pain subsides.
4. Apply one drop of lavender essential oil, neat, to each sting or bite.

Benefits:
Apple cider vinegar cleanses the sting or bite area and also affects the pH level of the area, which can combat the negative effects of wasp stings.

Roman chamomile and lavender essential oils are soothing and analgesic reducing both the pain and itching that occur with stings and bites. Lavender essential oil also has antimicrobial properties.

Rosemary essential oil cleanses the bite or sting area to prevent infection. It also has antimalarial properties.

Notes and Tips:
For children between the ages of three months and two years, follow the instructions above, but omit the rosemary essential oil and dilute the lavender essential oil with carrier oil.

For children over the age of two, replace the rosemary essential oil with basil essential oil to maintain the cleansing properties.

If a child's bite or sting gets infected, take the child, immediately, to see a medical professional.

Digestive Health and Nutrition

NUTRIENT ABSORPTION BOOSTING CAPSULE

Eating nutritious food doesn't do you any good if you aren't absorbing the nutrients it provides. The same goes for taking vitamins. There are several ways to improve nutrient absorption, including taking probiotics, eating complementary foods, spacing meals, and taking the Nutrient Absorption Boosting Capsule.

Ingredients:
1 drop black pepper essential oil
1 drop clove essential oil
honey
vegetable capsule

Preparation and administration:
1. Open vegetable capsule.
2. Add 1 drop each of black pepper and clove bud essential oils.
3. Fill with honey.
4. Swallow with water.

Benefits:
Black pepper essential oil contains piperine which increases the bioavailability of nutrients in food.
Clove essential oil is an antioxidant. It increases the absorption of nutrients by reducing the oxidization of those nutrients in the gastrointestinal tract.

Notes and Tips:
Vegetable capsules do not hold essential oils for a long period of time. Take the Nutrient Absorption Boosting Capsule immediately upon preparation.

FOOD POISONING PREVENTION CAPSULE

Eating can be an adventure and sometimes part of that adventure comes with the risk of food poisoning. We don't always trust the source of our food, be it street vendor, food truck, foreign country, or even a high-end local restaurant, but that shouldn't prevent us from trying new food and exploring the culinary possibilities out there. Proper preparation of food at home is the best prevention of food poisoning, but when eating out—especially in less than sanitary situations—having a backup plan is the best precaution. This capsule filled with antimicrobial oils is the backup plan you need.

Most cases of food poisoning are mild, but still incredibly unpleasant. Food poisoning can be caused by bacteria, viruses, or parasites due to food spoilage, contamination, or improper food handling. The most common food-borne pathogens are noroviruses, *Campylobacter,* and *Salmonella.* Other food-borne pathogens that are of heightened concern are *Giardia lamblia, Escherichia coli,* and *Staphylococcus.* The essential oils in this blend are effective against this wide variety of food-borne pathogens.

Ingredients:
1 drop basil essential oil
1 drop cinnamon essential oil
1 drop clove essential oil
1 drop lemongrass essential oil
1 drop oregano essential oil
1 drop thyme essential oil
vegetable capsule

Preparation:
1. Open the vegetable capsule.
2. Add 1 drop each of basil, cinnamon, clove, lemongrass, and thyme essential oils.
3. Close the vegetable capsule.

Administration:
1. Swallow the vegetable capsule using the pill-taking method you would use for any medication or vitamins.

Benefits:

Oregano essential oil destroys the RNA of the norovirus.

Cinnamon essential oil is prized for its antibacterial properties. In multiple studies, *Salmonella* has been found to be highly susceptible to cinnamon essential oil. Along with clove and thyme essential oils, cinnamon essential oil also inhibits *Campylobacter, Escherichia coli, Staphylococcus,* and *Listeria monocytogenes.*

Basil essential oil has been used in traditional medicine to treat a variety of gastrointestinal distresses. Basil essential oil, due to its high linalool content, is particularly effective against *Giardia lamblia.*

Lemongrass essential oil is antiparasitic. Parasites are less common than bacteria in food, but they are still a debilitating food-borne pathogen, which you want to avoid. Lemongrass is also antibacterial against *e. coli* and *Salmonella.*

Notes and Tips:

Using a fat-containing liquid—such as 2% or whole milk or a smoothie, to take the capsule—instead of water—will help dissolve the essential oils in your digestive tract. Essential oils are hydrophobic and do not dissipate in water.

An alternative method for taking the capsule is to place it in a spoonful of full-fat yogurt and swallow the capsule that way. If you eat a full serving of yogurt, you receive the added benefits of the probiotics, which improve your digestive health.

STOMACH BUG BOMB

There are a wide variety of stomach "bugs," none of which are actually caused by bugs. Instead, they are caused by bacteria, viruses, fungi, and parasites. These "bugs" can be passed from person to person, contracted from contaminated surfaces, or ingested in food or drinks. No matter how we catch a stomach "bug," we want to recover from it fast. As soon as you start to feel that queasy feeling in your stomach, take the Stomach Bug Bomb to expedite a quicker recovery.

Ingredients:

1 tablespoon raw honey
1 large crushed garlic clove
1 drop basil essential oil
1 drop black pepper essential oil
1 drop cinnamon essential oil
1 drop ginger essential oil
1 drop lemongrass essential oil

Preparation:

1. Use the flat side of a butter knife or a garlic press to crush 1 large clove of garlic.
2. Place the crushed clove of garlic in a large metal spoon.
3. Pour 1 tablespoon raw honey over the garlic clove.
4. Add 1 drop each of basil, black pepper, cinnamon, ginger, and lemongrass essential oils.

Administration:

1. Place the entire contents of the spoon into your mouth.
2. Chew the crushed garlic.
3. Swallow the Stomach Bug Bomb.

Benefits:

Raw honey and cinnamon essential oil are both antibiotic, killing bacteria that may be the cause of stomach infections.

Raw garlic is antiparasitic, specifically against *Giardia, Trypanosoma, Leishmania,* and *Plasmodium.*

Lemongrass essential oil is antibacterial and antiparasitic with a particular capacity against *Trypanosoma.*

Basil, cinnamon, and ginger essential oils are all effective against *Giardia.*

Black pepper essential oil has the ability to affect the cellular membranes of bacteria, causing them to break down. It's effective against both gram positive and gram negative bacteria including *Staphylococcus aureus, Bacillus cereus, Streptococcus faecalis, Pseudomonas aeruginosa, Salmonella typhi,* and *Escherichia coli.*

Orégano essential oil is highly antiviral.

Notes and Tips:
CAUTION: Lemongrass and oregano essential oils can be irritating to the lips. Applying lip balm before ingesting this blend protects your lips from irritation.

Prevent stomach "bugs" by taking the Food Poisoning Prevention Capsules (page 46).

DIARRHEA CALMING PROTOCOL

Other than the childhood song on the topic, diarrhea is not often brought up, despite how common an ailment it is. Diarrhea is one of the leading causes of death in the world and a serious symptom of many diseases. The food we eat, the stress in our lives, and the mere act of interacting with other people can all lead to diarrhea. Most cases of diarrhea are not life threatening, but the sooner it is addressed, the less likely it is to become a major problem. The Diarrhea Calming Protocol soothes the gastrointestinal system, allowing it to work properly to mitigate fluid loss.

DIARRHEA CALMING TEA
Ingredients:
10 ounces water
1 chamomile tea bag
1 lemon balm tea bag
2 tablespoons raw honey
1 drop ginger essential oil
1 drop lemon essential oil
1 drop peppermint essential oil

Preparation and administration:
1. Heat 10 ounces of water to just below a simmer.
2. Pour the hot water into a ceramic or tempered glass mug.
3. Add 1 bag each of chamomile and lemon balm tea.
4. Allow to steep for 5 minutes.
5. Remove tea bags.
6. Mix in 2 tablespoons of raw honey.

7. Add 1 drop each of ginger, lemon, and peppermint essential oils.
8. Sip leisurely until you have consumed the entire Diarrhea Calming Tea.

DIARRHEA CALMING CAPSULE
Ingredients:
vegetable capsule
6 drops black pepper essential oil
2 drops peppermint essential oil
2 drops chamomile essential oil
2 drops fennel essential oil
coconut oil

Preparation and administration:
1. Open vegetable capsule.
2. Add 6 drops black pepper essential oil and 2 drops each of peppermint, chamomile, and fennel essential oils.
3. Top with coconut oil.
4. Close capsule.
5. Take capsule with water, coconut water, or coconut milk.

DIARRHEA CALMING MASSAGE BLEND
Ingredients:
1 teaspoon sweet almond oil (or other carrier oil)
3 drops chamomile essential oil
2 drops orange essential oil
1 drop ginger essential oil

Preparation and administration:
1. Remove caps from essential oils.
2. Pour 1 teaspoon sweet almond essential oil into the palm of your hand.
3. Add 3 drops chamomile, 2 drops orange, and 1 drop ginger essential oils to your palm.
4. Rub the blend of oils over your entire abdomen.
5. Recap essential oils.

Benefits:
Diarrhea is often accompanied by feelings of nausea. Ginger essential oil soothes this nausea and is in and of itself antidiarrhetic.

Peppermint essential oil is particularly helpful with irritable bowel syndrome, which often results in spasmodic diarrhea. By reducing the spasms in the intestines, peppermint essential oil regulates the flow of digestion, allowing time for the proper absorption of fluid from the stools.

Chamomile is also antispasmodic, calming the stomach and intestines.

Black pepper contains constituents including piperine, which have both spasmodic and antispasmodic properties. This allows black pepper essential oil to aid the intestines in the appropriate speed of digestion.

Orange essential oil reduces the perception of feelings of pain associated with diarrhea, but most importantly it relieves stress, which can contribute to gastrointestinal distress.

Lemon Balm—a.k.a. Melissa—is great for reducing stress.

Fennel has been historically used—from ancient India, Greece, and Rome to colonial America—to aid in digestive health.

Notes and Tips:

The Diarrhea Calming Massage Blend is safe for children over the age of two. For children under the age of two simply use chamomile essential oil diluted to a 0.5 percent dilution.

Peppermint essential oil can cause acid reflux when ingested directly (as opposed to in a capsule), but the lemon essential oil reduces acid reflux due to its gastroprotective qualities.

CONSTIPATION RELIEF PROTOCOL

Constipation, like diarrhea, is not something we talk about in polite company, but is an issue affecting almost everyone at some point in their lives. Diet plays a huge role in digestive health, especially in relation to constipation. Eating fibrous and probiotic foods, plus drinking plenty of water are the first defenses against constipation. However, this is not always enough to keep the bowels moving. Hereditary conditions, diseases, and medications all play a part in disrupting the movement of your bowels. When your bowels are clogged, use the recipes in the Constipation Relief Protocol to restore your digestive flow.

CONSTIPATION RELIEF CAPSULE
Ingredients:
castor oil
1 drop basil essential oil
1 drop fennel essential oil
1 drop oregano essential oil
1 drop peppermint essential oil
vegetable capsule

Preparation and administration:
1. In a vegetable capsule, combine 1 drop each of basil, fennel, oregano, and peppermint essential oils.
2. Fill the rest of the capsule with castor oil.
3. Close the vegetable capsule.
4. Immediately after filling, swallow the Constipation Relief Capsule with 8 ounces of room temperature water.

CONSTIPATION RELIEF TEA
Ingredients:
2–4 teaspoons castor oil
2 drops ginger essential oil
8 ounces water

Preparation and administration:
1. Heat 8 ounces of water to a drinkable, yet hot, temperature.
2. Add 2–4 teaspoons of castor oil into a ceramic or insulated glass teacup or coffee mug. Note: start with 2 teaspoons of castor oil and increase amount daily until constipation is relieved.
3. Add 2 drops ginger essential oil to the castor oil.
4. Pour the 8 ounces of heated water into the teacup/coffee mug.
5. Drink the entire Constipation Relief Tea immediately after preparation.

CONSTIPATION RELIEF MASSAGE BLEND
Ingredients:
1 tablespoon castor oil
6 drops rosemary essential oil

4 drops lemon essential oil

2 drops peppermint essential oil

Preparation and administration:
1. Open the essential oil bottle caps.
2. Pour 1 tablespoon castor oil into the palm of your hand.
3. Add 6 drops rosemary, 4 drops lemon, and 2 drops peppermint essential oils.
4. Rub the blend in a clockwise direction over your abdomen.
5. Recap your essential oils.

CONSTIPATION RELIEF REFLEXOLOGY BLEND
Ingredients:
1 tablespoon castor oil

8 drops basil essential oil

2 drops oregano essential oil

Preparation and administration:
1. In a small glass bowl, pour 1 tablespoon castor oil.
2. Add 8 drops of basil and 2 drops of oregano essential oil.
3. Mix oils together with a metal or wooden spoon or chopstick.

Administration:
1. Dip the tips of your fingers in the Constipation Relief Reflexology Blend.
2. Use your fingertips to massage the area between the narrowest part of the arch of your foot and your heel on each foot. Make sure to massage the inner arch and area along the outer exterior. Re-dip your fingers as needed while massaging.
3. Pour the remaining reflexology blend into the palm of your hand.
4. Rub your hands together and rub the blend into both your shins.

Benefits:
The use of fennel to aid digestion began thousands of years ago in India with Ayurvedic practitioners. This practice moved west, was recommended by the Greek and Roman physicians Hippocrates, Dioscorides, and Pliny

the Elder, introduced to central and northern Europe by Charlemagne, and brought even farther west to the Americas by European colonists.

Ginger and castor oil are also used in Ayurvedic medicine to treat constipation.

Topical and internal uses of basil essential oil aid digestion and relieve constipation.

Peppermint essential oil soothes irritable bowels by reducing inflammation. This allows the bowels to relax and let fecal matter pass.

Stomach massage with rosemary, lemon, and peppermint essential oil helps to move the bowels, facilitating the excretion of feces. Rubbing in a clockwise direction stimulates the bowels in the direction the contents of the colon travel.

Oregano is stomachic, improving the function of the stomach, which in turn improves digestive functioning.

In reflexology, the arch of the foot is connected to the digestive system. The area between the narrowest part of the foot and the heel specifically contain reflexes for the intestines.

Notes and Tips:

Drinking the Cleansing Water (page 56) will hydrate you—an important part of digestive health—along with promoting a cleansing of the intestines—also an important part of digestive health.

Enemas are the next step in the treatment of constipation. If complete constipation lasts for more than three days, use an enema. If that does not work, see your physician.

CAUTION: Oregano is considered a "hot" essential oil. Proper dilution with a carrier oil is important when using this essential oil.

LACTOSE INTOLERANCE SUPPORT

The best remedy for lactose intolerance is avoiding all dairy products, but that isn't always possible or enjoyable. Ice cream, cheese, smoothies, cream-based sauces, and other dairy filled foods are tempting and delicious. Not being able to enjoy these foods without digestive discomfort is frustrating. The two recipes included here for lactose intolerance support can be used before or after consuming dairy to aid digestion and soothe the symptoms of lactose intolerance.

LACTOSE INTOLERANCE PREVENTION CAPSULE
Ingredients:

1 drop lemongrass essential oil

honey

vegetable capsule

Preparation:
1. Open vegetable capsule.
2. Add one drop of lemongrass essential oil.
3. Fill the rest of the capsule with honey.
4. Close vegetable capsule.

Administration:
1. Swallow capsule with water or other nondairy drink.

LACTOSE INTOLERANCE STOMACH RUB
Ingredients:

1 drop lemongrass essential oil

1 teaspoon almond oil

Preparation:
1. Pour 1 teaspoon almond oil into the palm of your hand.
2. Add one drop of lemongrass essential oil.

Administration:
1. Rub mixture over your abdomen—in a clockwise motion—focusing on the stomach and small intestines.

Benefits:

Lemongrass essential oil is traditionally used in Brazilian and Southeast Asian medicine to treat gastrointestinal issues. It controls diarrhea—which is often a symptom of lactose intolerance—and its anti-inflammatory properties soothe the intestinal lining that is irritated by the consumption of dairy products by someone with lactose intolerance.

Honey has also been used since ancient times to treat gastrointestinal issues. Ancient Arab and Roman societies used honey to prevent diarrhea and modern research has substantiated this practice. Honey is well known for its anti-inflammatory properties.

Notes and Tips:

The Lactose Intolerance Prevention Capsule may be used in children over the age of six. The Lactose Intolerance Stomach Rub is safe, with proper dilution, for children over the age of two years old.

When using the Lactose Intolerance Stomach Rub for children, instead of the capsule, a teaspoon of honey taken orally will give additional anti-inflammatory benefits and prevent diarrhea.

Lemongrass essential oil can be irritating to the skin. This is why the dilution rate in this recipe is 1 percent. However, if you still find that this amount of dilution irritates your skin, use two teaspoons of almond oil.

HANGOVER RELIEF PROTOCOL

No one plans to have a hangover, but sometimes the day after you've indulged, you wake up with a pounding headache, sour stomach, and a general feeling of malaise. You may have only had a single glass of cheap champagne or so much to drink that the ill feelings began the night before—but no matter the cause, the result remains unpleasant. While standard preventative measures like moderation, hydration, and eating properly can help, they don't always work. However, with this hangover relief protocol, you can soothe that headache, calm that stomach, and give yourself the energy to get out of bed the next day.

The recipes needed for this protocol are listed first. Since we don't always plan ahead, these recipes can be made in advance to have on hand—or made as you need them. The protocol for using the recipes and additional essential oils is divided into three parts: before drinking, after drinking, and upon waking.

CLEANSING WATER (USED IN ALL STAGES)
Ingredients:

16 ounces of water

2 drops lemon essential oil

Preparation (at the time of use):

1. In a pint-size glass, pour 16 ounces of water.
2. Add 2 drops lemon essential oil.

DETOXIFYING BLEND (USED IN ALL STAGES)
Ingredients:

1 tablespoon sweet almond oil

2 drops lemon essential oil

2 drops thyme essential oil

2 drops cilantro essential oil

2 drops rosemary essential oil

Preparation:

1. In a ½-ounce (15 mL) blue or amber glass bottle, mix 1 tablespoon almond oil with 2 drops each of lemon, thyme, rosemary, and cilantro essential oils.
2. Cap the bottle tightly and shake to mix.
3. Use, or store for later in a cool, dry, and dark location.

NAUSEA-SOOTHING BLEND (USED IN THE LAST TWO STAGES OF THIS PROTOCOL)
Ingredients:

1 tablespoon sweet almond oil

1 drop ginger essential oil

1 drop fennel essential oil

1 drop clove essential oil

1 drop peppermint essential oil

Preparation:

1. In a ½-ounce (15 mL) blue or amber glass bottle, mix 1 tablespoon almond oil with 1 drop each of ginger, fennel, clove, and peppermint essential oils.
2. Cap the bottle tightly and shake to mix.
3. Use, or store for later in a cool, dry, and dark location.

BLOODY MARY RECIPE
Ingredients:

1 drop lime essential oil

1 drop black pepper essential oil

1 cup tomato-based vegetable juice

1 ounce vodka (optional)
1 tablespoon pickle juice
1 teaspoon olive brine
a dash of Worcester sauce
ice
a pinch of celery salt
1 stalk of celery
1 dill pickle spear
2 garlic-stuffed olives

Preparation:

1. Fill a martini shaker halfway with ice and add 1 drop lime essential oil, 1 drop black pepper essential oil, 1 cup tomato-based vegetable juice, 1 ounce vodka (optional), 1 tablespoon pickle juice, 1 teaspoon olive brine, a dash of Worcester sauce.
2. Shake.
3. Strain into a 16-ounce glass filled with ice and garnish with 1 pickle spear, 2 garlic stuffed olives, 1 celery stalk, and a pinch of celery salt.
4. Drink immediately or store in the refrigerator.

Before drinking:
Ingredients:
Cleansing Water
1 teaspoon of detoxifying blend

Protocol:

1. Drink entire glass of cleansing water.
2. Rub 1 teaspoon of the detoxifying blend over your liver.
3. Cap the glass bottle and save the remaining blend for later.

After drinking:
Ingredients:
Cleansing Water
1 teaspoon of detoxifying blend
1 teaspoon of nausea-soothing blend

Protocol:

1. Drink entire glass of cleansing water.
2. Apply 1 teaspoon of the detoxifying blend over your liver.
3. Apply 1 teaspoon of the nausea-soothing blend over your stomach and intestines.
4. Go to sleep.

Upon waking:
Ingredients:

cleansing water
2 teaspoons of sweet almond oil, divided evenly
1 drop peppermint essential oil
1 drop rosemary essential oil
1 teaspoon of detoxifying blend
2 teaspoons of nausea-soothing blend, divided evenly
Bloody Mary

Protocol:

1. Drink entire glass of cleansing water.
2. Put 1 teaspoon of sweet almond oil in the palm of your hand and add one drop of peppermint oil.
3. Rub your hands together and massage your temples (away from your eyes), forehead, and the base of your skull with the diluted peppermint essential oil to soothe and cool your headache. Be careful to avoid getting any of this mixture in your eyes.
4. Put the other teaspoon of sweet almond oil in your palm and add 1 drop of rosemary essential oil.
5. Rub your hands together and massage your scalp and the base of your skull with the diluted rosemary oil to reduce feelings of malaise.
6. Apply 1 teaspoon of the detoxifying blend over your liver.
7. Apply 1 teaspoon of the nausea-soothing blend over your stomach and intestines.
8. Make and drink the Bloody Mary recipe.
9. If nausea returns, use the remaining teaspoon of nausea-soothing blend.

Benefits:

The limonene in lemon and lime essential oils help your liver's detoxification process by stimulating it to produce detoxifying enzymes that flush both the limonene and other foreign toxins, including alcohol, from your body. By consuming lemon essential oil before you begin drinking alcohol, your body is prepared to process the alcohol immediately.

Thyme, rosemary, and black pepper essential oils all have antioxidant properties that help protect your liver from damage. Black pepper essential oil also helps reduce cravings for alcohol the next day.

Ginger essential oil soothes feelings of nausea.

Fennel and clove essential oils both aid in digestion and the analgesic properties of clove oil can calm an upset stomach and intestines.

Notes and Tips:

A nonalcoholic Bloody Mary is more conducive to recovering from a hangover, but some people find that a small amount of alcohol the next morning helps them. Not including the vodka in the Bloody Mary recipe is recommended.

The Bloody Mary recipe can be made the night before, but will not last longer than 24 hours in the refrigerator.

If stored properly in a cool, dry, and dark location, the detoxifying blend and nausea-soothing blend with maintain efficacy for at least a month.

Continue to drink water while imbibing liquor, beer, wine, or other alcoholic beverages. I advise one glass of water for every alcoholic drink.

Eat food before, and while, consuming alcohol.

Using the mouthwash provided in the oral hygiene section of this book will prevent tooth damage from the sugars present in alcoholic beverages.

The lotion bar in the self-care sections of this book will help with skin dehydration that can come with a hangover.

Mental Health

ANXIETY-RELIEVING HAND MASSAGE

We have all felt anxious at one time or another, whether it was anxiety over an upcoming event or a major life change. Frequent anxiety can increase the stress in our lives, leading to health and emotional concerns. Managing anxiety can come in many forms, including breathing techniques, exercise, yoga, medications, taking up a hobby, reading, therapy, and even spending time with friends and family. This essential oil hand massage can support a sense of well-being in conjunction with other anxiety-management techniques. Having a trusted friend, family member, or romantic partner administer this hand massage is the most effective way to reap the benefits because of the added positive effect of human interaction and skin-to-skin contact. However, you can also give this hand massage to yourself as form of personal wellness and care.

Ingredients:
1 teaspoon sweet almond oil
1 drop bergamot essential oil
1 drop lavender essential oil
1 drop frankincense essential oil

Preparation:
1. Pour 1 teaspoon of sweet almond oil into the palm of your hand or the hand of the person receiving the massage. Add one drop each of bergamot, lavender, and frankincense essential oils. Rub hands together to mix the oils and evenly distribute the massage oil.

Administration:
1. Begin with the hand facing up. Cradle the back of the hand with your fingers and place the pad of your thumb just below the pinky finger, opposite the base knuckle. With light pressure, rub in a circular motion slowly moving up a pinky finger all the way to tip. Spend a little extra

time massaging the tip of the finger. Repeat this process on each finger of the hand, including the thumb.

2. Turn the hand over and massage down the bones in the hand from the wrist to the fingertips.
3. Use the tips of your fingers to massage the space between each finger.
4. With long, sweeping motions, use your palm and fingers to massage up and down the forearm from the wrist to the elbow several times. Turn the hand back over and repeat on the underside of the forearm.
5. Find the tendons in the center of the wrist and use the pad of the thumb to massage between them in a circular motion.
6. With the palm now facing up, place your thumb in the center of the palm and massage in an outward spiral toward the thumb. End just below the hand between the tendons and the wrist bone (opposite the thumb).
7. Apply firm pressure to this point and then massage with a small circular motion.
8. Repeat with the other hand.

Benefits:

Bergamot essential oil subdues your heart rate, while lavender essential oil lowers blood pressure. Together bergamot and lavender essential oils have a synergistic effect and they work better in combination than alone. The addition of frankincense essential oil helps to mitigate the depression aspect of anxiety.

Notes and Tips:

After receiving this hand massage, inhale the scent of the massage oil blend to receive added aromatherapy benefits of these essential oils.

Some people are sensitive to the scent of lavender and would prefer to omit the lavender essential oil. This recipe and massage can still be beneficial without the lavender essential oil.

When administering this massage to yourself, it can be helpful to take the caps off of the essential oils before you put the almond oil in your palm. Make sure to reapply the caps as soon as you have rubbed the oil into your hands (before you begin the massage) so that the essential oils do not begin to evaporate.

Bergamot essential oil can cause sun sensitivities, so be cautious when going out in the sun for up to twelve hours after using this massage oil.

The amount of sweet almond oil can be increased for those with skin sensitivities. This will not reduce the efficacy of the essential oils.

STRESS-RELIEVING DIFFUSER BLEND

Stress is a part of life, but too much stress has serious consequences for our health and well-being. Continuously high stress levels are leading causes of heart disease, stroke, inflammatory diseases, premature aging, and getting sick in general. Stress can come in many forms—including work, family, and emotional and financial distress—but no matter the cause, there are ways to deal with stress in a healthy manner. The Stress-Relieving Diffuser Blend helps your body mitigate the effects of stress and your mind feel at peace.

Ingredients:
½ cup water
4 drops lavender essential oil
3 drops bergamot essential oil
2 drops lemon essential oil

Preparation:
1. Add ½ cup of water (or the amount recommended by your diffuser) to the well of your diffuser.
2. Add 4 drops of lavender essential oil, 3 drops of bergamot essential oil, and 2 drops lemon essential oil to the water.

Administration:
1. Place your diffuser on your desk at work or in the bathroom when you are taking a stress-relieving bath or shower—or wherever you are when you need some stress relief!
2. Turn on your diffuser and let the room fill with the relaxing aroma.
3. Take several deep breaths and then continue to breath normally.

Benefits:

Lavender essential oil reduces blood pressure and is commonly used for relaxation and stress relief.

Bergamot essential oil has been found to alleviate stress levels in students, teachers, and medical patients. Its uplifting qualities counterbalance the sedative properties of lavender, so you won't find yourself drifting off at work.

Lemon essential oil, like other citrus oils, is uplifting and stress reducing. The limonene and citral found in lemon essential oil inhibit the levels of stress hormones in the brain, reducing the mental and physical effects of stress.

Notes and Tips:

Combining this Stress-Relieving Diffuser Blend with your favorite relaxing music can amplify its effects. Music helps relieve stress, and the combination of olfactory and auditory stress relief has a synergistic effect, which increases the efficacy of both forms of stress relief.

BAD DAY BETTER DIFFUSER BLEND

We all have bad days. Some bad days are plain old bad days, while others are plain awful. Fights with our friends or family members, car accidents, parking tickets or fines of any kind, missed promotions or lost jobs, and just about any bad news can turn a perfectly pleasant day into a terrible one. When this happens it's time to pull out the big guns and ramp up the aromatherapy. The Bad Day Better Diffuser Blend pairs perfectly with your favorite book or movie and a good meal to turn a bad day into a better than average evening.

Ingredients:

½ cup water
6 drops bergamot essential oil
5 drops orange essential oil
4 drops ylang-ylang essential oil
4 drops frankincense essential oil
3 drops sandalwood essential oil
2 drops vetiver essential oil

Preparation:
1. Add ½ cup of water (or the amount recommended by your diffuser) to the well of your diffuser.
2. Add 6 drops bergamot essential oil, 5 drops orange essential oil, 4 drops ylang-ylang essential oil, 4 drops frankincense essential oil, 3 drops sandalwood essential oil, 2 drops vetiver essential oil to the water.

Administration:
1. Place your diffuser within four feet of yourself.
2. Turn on your diffuser and let the room fill with the relaxing aroma.
3. Take several deep breaths and then continue to breath normally.

Benefits:
Bergamot essential oil alleviates stress levels in students, teachers, and medical patients. Its uplifting qualities counterbalance the sedative properties of lavender, so you won't find yourself drifting off at work.

Orange essential oil is sometimes called "the happy oil" because it brings happiness to the brain and central nervous system.

Ylang-ylang essential oil elicits a sense of peace when inhaled.

Frankincense is an incredibly versatile essential oil. It improves mood and reduces the physiological effects of stress on the body.

Sandalwood is a meditative essential oil that brings balance to your mind and body.

Vetiver essential oil provides an aromatic and psychological base for this blend. It is a long-lasting and viscous essential oil that brings about a sense of euphoria.

Notes and Tips:
If you have time—before you collapse under the weight of your bad day—blending the essential oils before adding them to the diffuser will create a more uniform aroma and blend the vetiver essential oil more evenly with the other essential oils.

You can make make a larger batch of this blend (up to 8 times the amounts given in this recipe) and store the blend in a 15mL blue, green, or glass amber bottle. Just add 24 drops of the blend to your diffuser to get the same effect as adding the essential oils individually.

MEMORY ENHANCING PROTOCOL

Smell is the most powerful of the senses when it comes to memory, and it plays an important role in our learning process. We recognize our mother's scent before we recognize her voice or her face. If our partners are away, we nuzzle their pillows to stimulate positive memories about them. When we walk into a familiar place, it is the smells that greet us first. Certain smells can surprise us by bringing us back to a time or place we had almost forgotten, but recall immediately when an aroma associated with that time or place wafts by us. Using aromatherapy when learning new information or trying to take information already presented to us and solidify it into our long-term memory—a.k.a. studying—makes the process easier and more effective.

STUDY TIME DIFFUSER BLEND
Ingredients:
½ cup water
5 drops orange essential oil
3 drops rosemary essential oil
2 drops peppermint essential oil
1 drop eucalyptus essential oil

Preparation:
1. Fill your diffuser with ½ cup water—or the appropriate amount for your type of diffuser.
2. Add 5 drops orange, 3 drops rosemary, 2 drops peppermint, and 1 drop eucalyptus essential oils to the water.
3. If your diffuser has a top portion that needs to be replaced before using, place the top on now.

Administration:
1. Place your diffuser near where you will be while studying or learning new information.
2. Turn your diffuser on.
3. Inhale the aroma of the essential oils while you study or learn new information.

MEMORY CONSOLIDATION DIFFUSER BLEND

Ingredients:

½ cup water

5 drops lavender essential oil

3 drops orange essential oil

Preparation:

1. Fill your diffuser with ½ cup water—or the appropriate amount for your type of diffuser.
2. Add 5 drops lavender and 3 drops orange essential oils to the water.
3. If your diffuser has a top portion that needs to be replaced before using, place the top on now.

Administration:

1. Place your diffuser next to your bed.
2. After studying, or learning new information, turn the diffuser on as you fall asleep to consolidate the information you learned into your mind and to make the information more accessible later.
3. Continue to diffuse the blend while you sleep.

MEMORY RECALL BLEND FOR AROMATHERAPY PENDANT

Ingredients:

1 drop rosemary essential oil

2 drops orange essential oil

Preparation:

1. Add 1 drop of rosemary essential oil and 2 drops of orange essential oil to an aromatherapy pendant.

Administration:

1. Wear your aromatherapy while taking a test or in a situation where you are trying to recall the information you were learning while using the Study Time Diffuser Blend.
2. When you are struggling to recall a particular bit of information, inhale deeply from the pendant.

Benefits:

Peppermint and eucalyptus essential oils stimulate your mind and keep you awake while studying.

Rosemary essential oil increases cognitive function and memory recall.

Using orange essential oil while studying, sleeping, and during test taking allows the process of learning and recalling information to flow naturally through olfactory stimulation. Orange essential oil will help relax your mood while you are learning new information. By reducing your anxiety about the studying or learning process, you are better able to absorb the information you are focused on. At the same time, the orange essential oil is preparing you to trigger an ability to access that information at a later point by creating an association between the smell of orange and that particular information. While sleeping, lavender and orange essential oils will consolidate the information you learned while you were awake. When you are trying to recall information that you learned while using the Study Time Diffuser Blend, the aroma of orange, from the Memory Recall Aromatherapy Blend, will trigger a powerful memory response linked to your study session.

Notes and Tips:

There are multiple styles of aromatherapy pendants available: metal pendants with cotton pads, glass pendants with corks, wooden pendants with wicks or for direct oil application, and clay pendants for direct oil application. The quality and style of your aromatherapy pendant will affect how often you need to reapply the Memory-Enhancing Aromatherapy Pendant Blend. Earth clay and wood pendants hold the essential oils the longest, which is ideal if your pendant is solely for use with this blend. However, if you want to change out your essential oil blend frequently, pendants with cotton pads give you this flexibility.

Orange essential oil is ideal for this protocol, but if you have multiple subjects you are studying over a relatively short period of time, you can substitute a different citrus oil for each subject to differentiate between the types of information you are trying to recall.

For an extra memory boost, use the Gentle Rosemary-Orange Shampoo included on page 135 in this book the morning of your test.

CREATIVITY-BOOSTING DIFFUSER BLEND

Creativity comes in many forms. The arts, humor, writing, business, parenting, friendships, dating, marriage, crafting, inventing, and life in general all require at least some degree of creativity. Life requires us to think outside the box, but also saps us of the energy needed to do so. When you need to access the part of your brain that expands beyond the everyday, use the Creativity-Boosting Diffuser Blend to tap your inner creativity.

Ingredients:
4 drops lemon essential oil
4 drops grapefruit essential oil
2 drops geranium essential oil
1 drop frankincense essential oil
1 drop vetiver essential oil
½ cup water

Preparation:
1. In a small glass bowl, add each of the essential oils in the order of the ingredient list. Swish the bowl around to gently blend the essential oils together.
2. Add ¼ cup of water to the bowl and swish the bowl around again to integrate the essential oils into the water. Add this mixture to a essential oil diffuser.
3. Add the remaining water to the bowl, swirl the water around to include any remaining essential oil left in the bowl, and pour into the diffuser.

Administration:
1. Place your diffuser in a central location that allows for you to move around in your space and still be able to inhale the aroma it will emit.
2. Follow the directions for the diffuser to diffuse the Creativity-Boosting Blend.

Benefits:
Lemon essential oil increases feelings of well-being and creativity.
Grapefruit essential, like other citrus essential oils, uplifts the mood.

Geranium essential oil reduces anxiety and anecdotal evidence claims that it encourages a healthy sense of humor.

Grapefruit and geranium essential oils stimulate the right side of the brain, which is linked to creativity.

Frankincense is a highly versatile essential oil that has a positive effect on the central nervous system. It aids memory, mood, and mental clarity. It also has spiritual and religious connections and connotations that promote its use in a creativity blend.

Vetiver essential oil is used to for focus and balance.

Notes and Tips:

The preparation of the essential oil blend prior to adding the essential oils to the diffuser is due to the high viscosity of vetiver oil. By mixing the vetiver oil with the lighter citrus oils first, the essential oil blend will be released more evenly from the diffuser. The viscosity of the vetiver essential oil also means that it takes longer for the a drop of vetiver essential oil to release from the bottle than multiple drops of the other essential oils.

If any of the oils in this blend elicit negative memory responses, replace them with similar oils or omit them entirely. Vetiver can be replaced by increasing the amount of frankincense or by substituting myrrh. Similarly, the frankincense essential oil can be replaced by myrrh essential oil. Lemon essential oil can be substituted by lime or orange essential oils and still maintain the recipe's sense of well-being. Like grapefruit essential oil, bergamot essential oil uplifts the mood and stimulates the right side of the brain. Therefore, it can be used to supplant the grapefruit essential oil. Neroli and rose essential oils are expensive, but suitable substitutes for the geranium essential oil in this recipe.

ROMANTIC MASSAGE BLEND

The thought of essential oils can conjure up images of a tent filled with colorful carpets, tapestries, scarves, and pillows; sensual music; and a romantic partner ready to give you a sensuous massage. Essential oils have long been prized as aphrodisiacs, and their ability to both relax and invigorate us make them ideal for use in the bedroom. A romantic massage brings intimacy to a relationship. This is especially important in long-term relationships, where the daily routine can interfere with the romantic bonds that are necessary to maintain a healthy partnership.

When using this romantic massage blend, don't forget to create a romantic mood with more than just essential oils. Light some unscented candles, create a visually appealing space, and get comfortable.

Ingredients:
sweet almond oil
8 drops ylang-ylang essential oil
4 drops clary sage essential oil
2 drops bergamot essential oil
2 drops sandalwood essential oil

Preparation:
1. Combine 8 drops ylang-ylang, 4 drops clary sage, 2 drops bergamot, and 2 drops sandalwood essential oils in a 1-ounce (15mL) blue or amber glass bottle.
2. Top with sweet almond oil.
3. Shake to combine ingredients.

Administration:
A sensual massage is very personal, and individual preferences vary greatly. It is important to listen to your partner's desires and to express your own desires as well. Therefore, instead of step-by-step instructions on giving a massage using the romantic massage blend, this section will include some suggested massage techniques to use with your partner.

Face massage:
Place a couple drops of the romantic massage blend onto the tips of your fingers. Lay your partner's head in your lap and gently stroke from the tip of the chin along the edge of the face to the forehead. Use the pads of your fingertips to stroke both cheeks. Run your fingers through your partner's hair. Use your thumb and pointer finger to gently rub the earlobe and outside edge of your partner's ears, going up and up and down several times. Use the tip of your ringer finger to gently touch the inner ridges of your partner's ears. Finish by stroking down on the earlobes.

Back massage:

Straddle your partner's lower back (do not place your weight on your partner) and pour several drops of the massage oil down your partner's spine. Use your flat hands to spread the oil out along your partner's back from the shoulders down to the base of the spine. Draw your fingers up the spine and blow in a circular motion on the back of your partner's neck. Continue the massage by starting at the base of the spine and fanning upward toward the shoulders.

Upper thighs and buttocks:

Drizzle a few drops of the romantic massage blend onto the back of your partner's thighs and buttocks. Use your pointer and middle fingers to rub the blend into the skin using circular motions. Then use your palms to knead the thighs and buttocks. Finish with a light brushing of the fingertips from the back of the knees up to the buttocks.

Chest, stomach, and pelvis:

Put a dime-size amount of the romantic massage blend into your palm and rub your hands together. Use circular motions to massage the blend into your partner's chest and abdomen. Reduce the pressure and use a feathery touch to make circular motions on your partner's pelvis.

Arms and inner thighs:

Place a couple of drops of the romantic massage blend on your fingertips and use a feathery touch to stroke the soft skin of the inner arms and thighs. Apply a little firmer pressure when stroking the tendons in the wrist or if your partner is ticklish. This part of a sensual massage is great for making eye contact.

Benefits:

The aromas in this massage stimulate the limbic system, which in turn plays a key role in sexuality.

Ylang-ylang essential oil has pheromonal properties and has been used as an aphrodisiac by ancient Egyptians including Cleopatra.

Clary sage is hormone balancing and an antidepressant. This improves your mood in the bedroom. It also has a gentle spasmodic effect on the uterus.

Bergamot essential oil is a mood stimulator and relieves anxiety. Anxiety is often a barrier to romantic interaction and the addition of bergamot essential oil addresses that.

Sandalwood essential oil acts as an aphrodisiac by increasing pulse rate, blood flow, and our perception of the attractiveness of others.

Notes and Tips:

Due to the sensitive connection between aroma and sexuality, you can adjust the intensity of the aroma in the blend by adjusting the ratio of essential oils to sweet almond oil. For a lighter aroma, include half the number of drops of each essential oil.

CAUTION: Bergamot essential oil can cause sun sensitivity. If using this blend before going out, uncovered, into the sun, wash the blend off using any of the bodywash recipes in this book.

Parenthood and Children

FERTILITY SUPPORT PROTOCOL

Fertility is an emotional topic for many people. These emotions include joy, fear, excitement, sadness, stress, elation, hope, and anticipation, just to name a few! Trying to conceive is an intimate affair, but with the variety of barriers that can make conception difficult—age, health, nutrition, environmental factors, genetics, etc.—there can be a much broader group involved in the process. Family, friends, health-care providers, and even strangers have advice and tools to provide a couple in the process of creating new life. This fertility protocol is not a magical cure-all that replaces the sound counsel of your doctor, nurse, or midwife. Instead, it is meant to be a tool to use in conjunction with the other tools provided to you. If you are working with health-care professionals to improve your chances of conception, make sure to review this protocol with them to confirm that there are not any contraindicating medications that would be affected by essential oils.

The recipes used in this protocol are listed first, with notes on when to use them. The Fertility Support Protocol itself is listed next and split into two main sections: for her and for him. It takes two people to make a baby, and both benefit from the use of essential oils to increase fertility. The two sections are then further broken down into stages based on your or your partner's menstrual cycle. Essential oils that considered spasmodic are omitted in the later sections of the protocol in case they might negatively affect uterine stability.

CLEANSING WATER (USED IN ALL STAGES)
Ingredients:
16 ounces water
2 drops lemon essential oil

Preparation and Administration:
1. Pour 16 ounces of water into a glass.
2. Add 2 drops lemon essential oil.
3. Drink immediately.

CLEANSING FERTILITY SUPPORT TEA (FOR HER: USED IN FIRST PART OF CYCLE)

Ingredients:

10 ounces water

1 chamomile tea bag

1 drop lemon essential oil

1 drop ginger essential oil

1 teaspoon manuka honey

Preparation and Administration:
1. Bring 10 ounces of water to a simmer.
2. Pour into a ceramic or tempered glass mug.
3. Add 1 chamomile tea bag.
4. Allow to steep for 5 minutes.
5. Remove tea bag.
6. Add 1 drop each of lemon and ginger essential oils.
7. (optional) Add 1 teaspoon manuka honey.
8. Drink tea.

CENTERING DROPS (USED IN ALL STAGES)

Ingredients:

2 drops avocado oil

2 drops frankincense essential oil

Preparation and Administration:
1. Place 2 drops of avocado oil under your tongue.
2. Add 2 drops of frankincense oil under your tongue.
3. Hold mixture under your tongue for 30 seconds.
4. Swallow.

BALANCING DROPS (USED IN ALL STAGES)

Ingredients:

10 drops avocado oil

10 drops grapefruit essential oil

Preparation and Administration:

1. Place 10 drops of avocado oil under your tongue.
2. Add 10 drops of grapefruit essential oil under your tongue.
3. Hold mixture under your tongue for 30 seconds.
4. Swallow.

PRE-CONCEPTION FERTILITY SUPPORT MASSAGE BLEND (USED IN FIRST TWO PARTS OF CYCLE)

Ingredients:

2 teaspoons avocado oil

4 drops clary sage essential oil

2 drops frankincense essential oil

2 drops geranium essential oil

2 drops myrrh essential oil

2 drops ylang-ylang essential oil

Preparation and Administration:

1. Take the caps off the avocado oil and essential oil bottles.
2. Pour 2 teaspoons avocado oil into your hand.
3. Add 4 drops clary sage, 2 drops frankincense, 2 drops myrrh, 2 drops ylang-ylang, and 2 drops geranium essential oils.
4. Rub your hands together to mix the oils.
5. Inhale aroma from your hands.
6. Massage into your lower abdomen, pelvis, and lower back.
7. Massage around your ankle bones (right ankle for her, left ankle for him).
8. Recap bottles.

UTERINE SUPPORT MASSAGE BLEND (USED IN THIRD PART OF CYCLE)

Ingredients:

2 teaspoons avocado oil

2 drops geranium essential oil

2 drops ylang-ylang essential oil

Preparation and Administration:

1. Take the caps off the avocado oil and essential oil bottles.

2. Pour 2 teaspoons avocado oil into your hand.
3. Add 2 drops each ylang-ylang and geranium essential oils.
4. Rub your hands together to mix the oils.
5. Inhale aroma from your hands.
6. Massage into your lower abdomen, pelvis, and lower back.
7. Massage around your ankle bones (right ankle for her, left ankle for him).
8. Recap bottles.

PRE-CONCEPTION LIVER SUPPORT MASSAGE BLEND (USED IN FIRST TWO PARTS OF CYCLE)
Ingredients:
1 teaspoon avocado oil
2 drops marjoram essential oil
2 drops thyme essential oil

Preparation and Administration:
1. Take the caps off the avocado oil and essential oil bottles.
2. Pour 1 teaspoon avocado oil into your hand.
3. Add 2 drops each marjoram and thyme essential oils.
4. Rub your hands together to mix the oils.
5. Inhale aroma from your hands.
6. Massage into your upper abdomen.
7. Recap bottles.

LIVER SUPPORT MASSAGE BLEND (USED IN THIRD PART OF CYCLE)
Ingredients:
1 teaspoon avocado oil
2 drops marjoram essential oil

Preparation and Administration:
1. Take the caps off the avocado oil and marjoram essential oil bottles.
2. Pour 1 teaspoon avocado oil into your hand.
3. Add 2 drops marjoram essential oil.
4. Rub your hands together to mix the oils.
5. Inhale aroma from your hands.

6. Massage into your upper abdomen.
7. Recap bottles.

OVARIAN SUPPORT MASSAGE BLEND (FOR HER: USED IN FIRST TWO PARTS OF CYCLE)
Ingredients:
½ teaspoon avocado oil (or other carrier oil)

2 drops chamomile essential oil

Preparation and Administration:
1. Take the caps off the avocado oil and chamomile essential oil bottles.
2. Pour ½ teaspoon avocado oil into your hand.
3. Add 2 drops chamomile essential oil.
4. Rub your hands together to mix the oils.
5. Inhale aroma from your hands.
6. Massage into your lower abdomen, specifically over the ovaries.
7. Recap bottles.

CIRCULATION SUPPORT MASSAGE BLEND (FOR HIM: USED IN FIRST PART OF CYCLE)
Ingredients:
½ teaspoon almond oil (or other carrier oil)

3 drops cypress essential oil

Preparation and Administration:
1. Take the caps off the avocado oil and cypress essential oil bottles.
2. Pour ½ teaspoon avocado oil into your hand.
3. Add 3 drops cypress essential oil.
4. Rub your hands together to mix the oils.
5. Inhale aroma from your hands.
6. Massage into your hands, feet, and lower abdomen.
7. Recap bottles.

ANTIMICROBIAL FOOT MASSAGE BLEND (USE IN FIRST PART OF CYCLE)
½ teaspoon avocado oil

1 drop oregano essential oil

Preparation and Administration:

1. Take the caps off the avocado oil and oregano essential oil bottles.
2. Pour ½ teaspoon avocado oil into your hand.
3. Add 1 drop oregano essential oil.
4. Rub your hands together to mix the oils.
5. Massage into the bottoms of your feet.
6. Recap bottles.

FERTILITY SUPPORT PROTOCOL FOR HER:

First part of cycle (starting on the first day of your menstrual cycle through day 10 of your cycle):

Morning: Drink Cleansing Water, use Centering Drops, and administer Pre-Conception Fertility Support Massage Blend.

Midday: Drink Cleansing Water and use Balancing Drops.

Evening: Drink Cleansing Fertility Support Tea. Administer Pre-Conception Liver Support Massage Blend, Ovarian Support Massage Blend, and Antimicrobial Foot Massage Blend.

Second part of cycle (Days 11–15):

Morning: Drink Cleansing Water, use Centering Drops, and administer Pre-Conception Fertility Support Massage Blend.

Midday: Drink Cleansing Water and use Balancing Drops.

Evening: Drink Cleansing Water. Administer Pre-Conception Liver Support Massage Blend and Ovarian Support Massage Blend.

Third part of cycle (Days 16–28):

Morning: Drink Cleansing Water, use Centering Drops, and administer Fertility Support Massage Blend.

Midday: Drink Cleansing Water and use Balancing Drops.

Evening: Drink Cleansing Water and administer Liver Support Massage Blend.

FERTILITY SUPPORT PROTOCOL FOR HIM:

First part of cycle (starting on the first day of her menstrual cycle through day 10 of her cycle):

Morning: Drink Cleansing Water, use Centering Drops, and administer Pre-Conception Fertility Support Massage Blend.

Midday: Drink Cleansing Water and use Balancing Drops.

Evening: Drink Cleansing Water. Administer Pre-Conception Liver Support Massage Blend, Circulation Support Massage Blend, and Antimicrobial Foot Massage Blend.

Second part of cycle (Days 11–15):

Morning: Drink Cleansing Water, use Centering Drops, and administer Pre-Conception Fertility Support Massage Blend.

Midday: Drink Cleansing Water and use Balancing Drops.

Evening: Drink Cleansing Water and administer Pre-Conception Liver Support Massage Blend.

Third part of cycle (Days 16–28):

Morning: Drink Cleansing Water, use Centering Drops, and administer Fertility Support Massage Blend.

Midday: Drink Cleansing Water and use Balancing Drops.

Evening: Drink Cleansing Water and administer Liver Support Massage Blend.

Benefits:

The reflexology points for the uterus and ovaries are in front of the ankle bones on the right foot.

The reflexology points for the prostate and testes are in front of the ankle bones on the left foot.

Lemon essential oil reduces stress, which can play a factor in fertility.

Prior alcohol use can damage the liver, which in turn can affect fertility.

Marjoram and thyme both contain antioxidants, which specifically improve liver and brain function along with fertility.

Grapefruit essential oil affects cortisol and progesterone levels in a manner that decreases stress and increases fertility.

Frankincense and myrrh essential oils can help with symptoms of endometriosis, fibroids, uterine strength, and inflammation, which may be affecting fertility.

Geranium essential oil is traditionally used in French aromatherapy to address sterility. It reduces stress and has antioxidant and antitumoral properties. It is particularly noted for its effect on uterine related tumors.

Clary sage and ylang-ylang essential oils are traditionally used in women's health because of their interaction with the endocrine system. They are especially important essential oils in relation to fertility. Clary sage is known to increase uterine contractions, which while this helps with conception, is a possibility of a negative effect on maintaining a pregnancy. Ylang-ylang, however, is generally recognized as safe for use during pregnancy.

Clary sage, ylang-ylang, and ginger essential oils all improve the libido.

Ylang-ylang is particularly soothing when absorbed through the skin.

Cypress essential oil improves circulation and blood flow, which is important for healthy sperm production.

Chamomile can reduce the symptoms of Polycystic Ovarian Syndrome (PCOS) and increase dominant follicles. It also helps to improve endometrial tissue arrangement. The antispasmolytic and anti-inflammatory properties of chamomile play a positive role in ovarian health and fertility.

Oregano essential oil is anti-infectious and will help clear the body of any lingering infections that may be inhibiting conception.

Manuka honey is used in Australian and New Zealand by Aborigines to treat wounds and other ailments due to its antimicrobial properties.

Avocado oil is high in vitamin E, which contributes to the elasticity of the skin and acts as an antioxidant.

Notes and Tips:
Use this Fertility Support Protocol for multiple cycles until conception occurs. Once conception has been confirmed or a menstrual cycle is missed, discontinue use.

Both partners should complete a cleanse for Candida albicans prior to attempting to conceive. Candida albicans may affect the ability of sperm to fertilize an egg.

Women trying to become pregnant or who are pregnant should vastly increase their water intake. Aim for a gallon of water per day. Besides increasing fertility and fetal health, staying hydrated reduces stretch marks.

Diet plays a huge role in fertility. Reduce your intake of sugars and processed foods. Increase your intake of green leafy vegetables along with fresh fruits and vegetables in general.

LABOR PROTOCOL

Delivering a child is a unique experience for every woman. Just as no pregnancy is the same, no birth is, either. There are a wide variety of birthing plans, and some parents don't make a plan at all. For some women, birth is a simple and relatively tolerable process. However, for others it is complicated and painful. Then, you have every combination between those ends of the spectrum. There are many interventions that can be used to reduce discomfort during childbirth, and each woman needs to choose what works best for her. This protocol is intended to calm, soothe, and reduce the pain and stress felt by women in labor.

AROMATHERAPEUTIC PAIN MANAGEMENT MASSAGE BLEND
Ingredients:
1 tablespoon grape-seed oil
4 drops lavender essential oil
3 drops geranium essential oil
2 drops Roman chamomile essential oil

Preparation:
1. Remove caps from oil bottles.
2. In the palm of the hand (this hand may belong to yourself, your partner, your doula, your midwife, your nurse, your friend, your mother, or anyone else you would like to be giving you a massage while you are in labor), pour 1 tablespoon grape-seed oil (or other carrier oil).

3. Add 4 drops lavender, 3 drops geranium, and 2 drops Roman chamomile.
4. Recap oil bottles.
5. Rub hands together to mix oils.

Administration:
Note: The administration of the Aromatherapeutic Pain Management Massage Blend depends on the type of pain felt by the laboring mother. There are two massage recommendations here, but other message methods can be employed as well. What is important is to listen to the needs of the laboring mother.

Massage for back pain:
1. Rub the Aromatherapeutic Pain Management Massage Blend around the lower back of the laboring mother.
2. Place hand where the mother feels the most discomfort.
3. Apply steady pressure to this area.

Effleurage for other labor pain:
1. Gently massage Aromatherapeutic Pain Management Massage Blend into the lower back of the laboring mother.
2. Use a featherlight touch to stroke the skin of the laboring mother.

LABOR RELAXATION DIFFUSER BLEND
Ingredients:
½ cup water
5 drops lavender essential oil
5 drops ylang-ylang essential oil
3 drops frankincense essential oil

Preparation and Administration:
1. Place your diffuser in a location where you will be able to smell the vapors, but not so close that it might be overwhelming or get knocked over.
2. Add ½ cup water (or amount recommended by the diffuser's instructions) to the diffuser.

3. Add 3 drops frankincense essential oil.
4. Add 5 drops each of lavender and ylang-ylang essential oil.
5. Plug the diffuser in and turn it on.
6. Refill as needed.

Benefits:

Effleurage stimulates the nerve endings and distracts from feelings felt by nerves in other parts of the body.

Receiving a massage during labor has been shown to reduce its duration.

Using aromatherapy during the birthing process has been found to reduce the need for other analgesics during labor. Aromatherapy can be used alone or in conjunction with additional analgesics.

Roman chamomile, lavender, ylang-ylang, geranium, and frankincense are all calming essential oils. They reduce stress and encourage relaxation. Stress, anxiety, and fear play a large role in the pain associated with labor, which in turn can lead to complications and the need for interventions. Reducing fear, pain, and stress promotes better outcomes for birthing mothers.

Roman chamomile essential oil reduces pain during labor. Roman chamomile is especially effective on back pain.

Geranium essential oil improves circulation and reduces blood pressure, which in turn improves breathing during labor.

Lavender works as a mild analgesic, as well as working within the brain to change the perception of pain. This means that even if your body is feeling pain, your mind is not registering it in the same way and the pain is more tolerable. This is especially helpful during the birthing process because laboring mothers need to focus on delivering their babies, not on their physical discomfort.

Like lavender, frankincense also reduces the perception of pain.

Aromatherapy using lavender essential oil has been shown to reduce the active phase and second stage of labor.

Notes and Tips:

Test the massage oil and diffuser blend before going into labor. You want to be sure the aromas are ones you find pleasant and relaxing. If any of the aromas are off-putting, exclude that essential oil from the recipe.

Make sure to ask those who are also attending the birth if they are comfortable with the aromas you will be using during labor and delivery.

BABY WASH

One joy of washing your infant is the beautiful scent of clean baby skin. A baby's bath is meant to be soothing and cleansing. Not every baby finds bath time as fun as others, but the lavender and Roman chamomile in the recipe soothe even fussy babies. Not only are lavender and Roman chamomile safe essential oils for children and babies, both have sedative qualities that can make bath time (and afterward) a calming experience for both parent and child. In fact, this wash is not just for babies—it's perfect for the whole family.

Ingredients:
1 cup unscented liquid Castile soap
¼ cup vegetable glycerin
8 drops lavender essential oil
4 drops Roman chamomile essential oil

Preparation:
1. Pour a ¼ cup vegetable glycerin into a small glass bowl.
2. Add 8 drops lavender essential oil and 4 drops Roman chamomile essential oil.
3. Mix with a metal spoon.
4. Pour this mixture into a 16-ounce blue or amber glass bottle, using a metal funnel.
5. Pour 1 cup unscented liquid Castile soap into the glass bottle, using the metal funnel.
6. Cap the bottle with a pump top.
7. Shake to mix.

Administration:
1. Shake essential oil before each use—the ingredients will naturally separate between uses.
2. Pump 2-3 pumps of baby wash onto a wet washcloth.

3. Gently rub the baby wash onto your child or baby's body and hair. Be careful to avoid the face, especially the eyes and mouth.
4. Rinse the baby wash off your child or baby thoroughly.

Benefits:

Lavender, long used to calm babies and help them sleep, is one of the few essential oils safe for nearly all ages—it's very gentle on skin.

Roman chamomile has sedative properties that can soothe skin and promote general relaxation.

Unscented Castile soap is not only gentle on babies' skin, it's free of harsh additives found in many commercial baby washes.

Glycerine is an emulsifier, helping to hold essential oils in the mixture without the risk of rancidity that can result when a carrier oil mixes with water.

Notes and Tips:

CAUTION: This baby wash is not intended for babies under the age of three months. Essential oils are not recommended on the sensitive skin of newborns.

COMFORTING DIAPER CREAM

Changing babies diapers regularly and keeping a baby's bottom dry are the best ways to prevent diaper rash, but sometimes that's not enough. Diaper rash can be painful for babies and toddlers, making diaper changes difficult and the whole family unhappy. The Comforting Diaper Cream soothes sore bottoms and prevents diaper rashes from occurring in the first place.

Ingredients:

½ cup virgin coconut oil
½ cup cornstarch
8 drops lavender essential oil
6 drops Roman chamomile essential oil
4 drops melaleuca essential oil (six months and older)

Preparation:

1. In a glass bowl, use an electric hand mixer to whip ½ cup solid virgin coconut oil until it makes peaks. This takes about 10 minutes depending on the weather.
2. Add 8 drops lavender and 6 drops Roman chamomile essential oils.
3. If your child is six months or older, add 4 drops melaleuca essential oil.
4. Mix until oils are evenly distributed.
5. Stir in ½ cup cornstarch. Mix until an even consistency is obtained.
6. Divide between 2–3 four-ounce mason jars.

Administration:

1. Using dry hands, scoop a small amount of Comforting Diaper Cream into your hand.
2. Gently rub onto your baby's clean, dry bottom.
3. Allow your baby to spend some time diaperless or put on a new diaper.

Benefits:

Coconut oil is soothing to the skin and protects against fungal infections, including candida infections.

Melaleuca essential oil is also effective against candida and other fungal infections.

Lavender and Roman chamomile essential oils are calming to the skin and relaxing for babies.

Lavender essential oil acts as a mild analgesic, reducing the pain babies feel when they have a diaper rash.

Cornstarch whisks moisture away from your baby's skin.

Notes and Tips:

Without melaleuca this recipe is safe for babies three months and above. With melaleuca, it is safe for children six months and above.

For a thicker consistency, add more cornstarch.

During hot weather, refrigerate your coconut oil before making this recipe so that the coconut oil begins in a solid state.

Store in a cool, dry location. During summer months, store in the refrigerator.

The Comforting Diaper Cream is safe for use with cloth or disposable diapers.

TANTRUM TAMING PROTOCOL

Tantrums occur when children—or even teenagers and adults—are tired, hungry, over stimulated, anxious, stressed, angry, or for seemingly absolutely no reason at all. Some tantrums begin slowly, with signs like agitation or whining, while others begin abruptly and completely out of the blue. No matter the cause or the buildup, parents and anyone who interacts with children know that tantrums are a part of being a child. No matter how well behaved the child, a tantrum is bound to occur at some (or many) points between discovering the development of wants, not just needs and adulthood. This Tantrum Taming Protocol provides several methods of dealing with tantrums at any point during the tantrum cycle.

Included in this protocol are two base blends: the Tantrum Taming Base and the Baby Calming Base. Both bases are meant to be made in advance so you have them on hand to use immediately. Having them available immediately allows you deal with the tantrum faster instead of having to put together an entire blend of oils while your child is midtantrum. These bases are the beginning of the other recipes in this protocol, which either can be put together midtantrum or made in advance. The Tantrum Taming Diffuser Blend and Massage Blend are presented with the preparation and administration together for the most efficient use of your time during a tantrum. The Tantrum Taming Sensory Dough can be made by yourself or with your child in advance and brought out before, during, or after a tantrum.

TANTRUM TAMING BASE (AGES 2 AND OVER)
Ingredients:

50 drops vetiver essential oil
30 drops ylang-ylang essential oil
30 drops bergamot essential oil
20 drops clary sage essential oil
20 drops marjoram essential oil
10 drops lavender essential oil
10 drops Roman chamomile essential oil
10 drops frankincense essential oil
10 drops sandalwood essential oil
10 drops cedarwood essential oil

Preparation:

1. In a 15 mL blue or amber glass bottle, combine 50 drops vetiver essential oil; 30 drops each of ylang-ylang and bergamot essential oils; 20 drops each of clary sage and marjoram essential oils; and 10 drops each of lavender, chamomile, frankincense, sandalwood, and cedarwood essential oils.
2. (Optional, but advised.) Place an orifice reducer into the mouth of the bottle. (Some caps come with the orifice reducer already in the cap for insertion when capping for the first time.)
3. Place the cap on the bottle. Tighten cap.
4. Shake well.

BABY CALMING BASE (6–23 MONTHS):

Ingredients:

30 drops bergamot essential oil
20 drops lavender essential oil
20 drops chamomile essential oil
10 drops sandalwood essential oil
10 drops cedarwood essential oil

Preparation:

1. In a 5 or 15 mL blue or amber glass bottle, combine 30 drops bergamot essential oil, 20 drops each of lavender and chamomile essential oils, and 10 drops each of sandalwood and cedarwood essential oils.
2. (Optional, but advised.) Place an orifice reducer into the mouth of the bottle. (Some caps come with the orifice reducer already in the cap for insertion when capping for the first time.)
3. Place the cap on the bottle. Tighten cap.
4. Shake well.

TANTRUM TAMING DIFFUSER BLEND

Ingredients:

½ cup water
10 drops Tantrum Taming Base or Baby Calming Base
4 drops bergamot essential oil

Preparation and Administration:

1. Add ½ cup water (or amount recommended by your diffuser instructions) to your diffuser.
2. Add 10 drops Tantrum Taming Base or Baby Calming Base and 4 drops bergamot essential to the water in the diffuser.
3. Turn diffuser on.
4. Encourage your child to inhale and then exhale with an extended out breath, while near the diffuser. If your child is too worked up to focus on breathing, just make sure the diffuser is within range of your child's ability to smell the Tantrum Taming Diffuser Blend.

TANTRUM TAMING MASSAGE BLEND:
Ingredients:

1 tablespoon solid raw coconut oil

8 drops Tantrum Taming Base or 4 drops Baby Calming Base (for children under 2)

2 drops grapefruit essential oil

Preparation and Administration:

1. Open the lids to your Tantrum Taming Base or Baby Calming Base and your grapefruit essential oil.
2. Tell your child that you want to show them something interesting.
3. Put 1 tablespoon solid raw coconut oil in the palm of your hand.
4. Have your child watch as the coconut oil melts from the heat of your hand.
5. Add 8 drops Tantrum Taming Base or 4 drops Baby Calming Base (for children under 2) and 2 drops grapefruit essential oil to the coconut oil in your palm.
6. Rub your hands together and massage your child's hands and/or feet with the Tantrum Taming Massage Blend. Pay special attention to the pads of the fingers and toes. (This is a great time to play "This Little Piggy.")
7. Massage any extra massage oil into the forearms and/or lower legs.
8. Allow your child to inhale the scent from your hands and inhale the scent yourself as well.

TANTRUM TAMING SENSORY DOUGH:

Ingredients:

2 cups water

2 cups flour

1 cup salt

1–2 tablespoons olive or coconut oil

2 teaspoons cream of tartar

3 drops Tantrum Taming Base or Baby Calming Base

3 drops orange essential oil

3 drops vanilla extract

food coloring (optional)

Preparation:

1. Pour 2 cups water into a large mixing bowl.
2. Add food coloring to reach desired color and intensity (optional).
3. Stir in dry ingredients (flour, salt, and cream of tartar).
4. Add 1 tablespoon olive or coconut oil and stir.
5. Pour contents of mixing bowl into a large pan/pot or onto a skillet and heat over medium heat.
6. Use a spatula to regularly stir the mixture until it forms a large ball.
7. Cool the ball of dough on parchment paper.
8. Once dough is cool, add 3 drops each of Tantrum Taming Base or Baby Calming Base, orange essential oil, and vanilla extract.
9. Knead dough to uniformly mix the oils and vanilla extract.
10. If the dough feels dry, add more olive or coconut oil until desired consistency is achieved.
11. Store dough in a glass jar in the refrigerator for several months or until it is no longer scented or easy to use.

Administration:

1. As soon as you notice your child headed toward a tantrum (you know the signs better than anyone else), take the Tantrum Taming Sensory Dough out of the refrigerator (or your bag) and give it to your child to play with.

Protocol Benefits:

Tantrums can be very stressful for children and are often brought on by stress. Vetiver essential oil reduces the effects of stress—both mentally and physically. Marjoram, lavender, and orange essential oils also help to relieve mental stress.

Vetiver, sandalwood, and grapefruit are euphoric essential oils that work with the hypothalamus and thalamus to allow the body to release hormones that regulate and improve mood. Essentially, these essential oils make your child happier.

Sandalwood essential oil lowers blood pressure and blinking rates (a sign of sedation) without making the user feel sedated. Using sandalwood essential oil actually increases a sense of focus and attentiveness. Sandalwood essential oil relaxes tired children without making them more tired.

Ylang-ylang essential oil also lowers blood pressure and improves mood. Both ylang-ylang and sandalwood essential oils work transdermally—through the skin—as well as through inhalation.

Bergamot essential oil is invigorating without being agitating. It reduces anxiety levels and gives children a sense of well-being. The addition of lavender and frankincense essential oils adds to the mood-enhancing properties of bergamot essential oil.

Clary sage essential oil works as an antistressor and antidepressant by modulating dopamine activity.

Cedarwood has traditionally been used by Native Americans. It is a sedative essential oil, which works on the nervous and respiratory systems.

Wild orange essential oil makes children feel less anxious. Anxiety can be both a cause and effect of a tantrum.

The inhalation of lavender and chamomile essential oil are traditional methods of relaxation.

Massage with and without essential oils decreases stress and relaxes both children and adults. Adding essential oils amplifies these effects.

Notes and Tips:

Do not use the Tantrum Taming Sensory Dough with children who usually eat their play dough. While the essential oils in the recipe are generally considered safe for ingestion, ingesting essential oils is not recommended for children under the age of 6. If your child does consume the dough, keep an eye on him/her for adverse reactions and seek medical attention if they occur.

SLEEPY TIME FOOT MASSAGE BLEND

Some days it's harder to get your child to sleep than others. A long, stimulating day can leave your child overstimulated, making it hard for the body to calm down and rest. Conversely, a day with too little activity can leave a child with extra energy to burn. No matter the cause of your child's sleeplessness, the Sleepy Time Foot Massage Blend will help you lull your child into sweet dreams.

Ingredients:
2 teaspoons sweet almond oil (or other carrier oil)
1 drop geranium essential oil
1 drop lavender essential oil
1 drop Roman chamomile essential oil
1 drop sandalwood essential oil

Preparation:
1. Remove caps from oil bottles.
2. Pour 2 teaspoons sweet almond oil into the palm of your hand.
3. Add 1 drop each geranium, lavender, Roman chamomile, and sandalwood essential oils.
4. Rub hands together.
5. Recap oil bottles.

Administration:
1. Massage child's feet with the Sleepy Time Foot Massage Blend.
2. Concentrate on your child's big toes and the arches of the feet.

Benefits:
Lavender, Roman chamomile, and sandalwood are all sedating essential oils.
Geranium essential oil is balancing.
The big toe is a sleep-inducing reflexology point.
Essential oils absorb well into the arch of the foot.

Notes and Tips:
This recipe is safe for babies and children ages six months and above.
   To make the Sleepy Time Foot Massage for adults, increase amount of essential oils to 3 drops each.

Speak soothingly to your child or sing a peaceful song while giving the Sleepy Time Foot Massage. This will encourage your child to relax and move into a mode of sleep.

A larger batch of this blend can be made and stored in a spray bottle to keep on hand for sleepless nights or middle of the night wake ups.

OWIE CALMING SPRAY

Part of growing up includes the requisite bumps and bruises that happen as children learn to balance, walk, and run; play on a daily basis; take risks; and have adventures. Sometimes, children pick back up, dust off, and keep going, but other times those scrapes, cuts, and bruises need a little extra care. This Owie Calming Spray disinfects, relieves pain, and calms emotions. Using this spray helps children feel better both physically and mentally. This spray is safe to use on children—and adults!—six months and above.

Ingredients:
30 drops lavender essential oil
30 drops melaleuca essential oil
10 drops frankincense essential oil
1.5 ounces witch hazel

Preparation:
1. In a 2-ounce blue or amber glass spray bottle, combine 30 drops each of lavender and melaleuca essential oils with 10 drops of frankincense essential oil.
2. Top with 1.5 ounces of witch hazel.
3. Apply spray cap tightly.
4. Shake well.

Administration:
If possible wash cuts and scrapes with soap and water before using. Otherwise, be sure to wipe away any dirt or debris with a clean cloth or tissue.
1. Shake before using.

2. Spray Owie Calming Spray directly on any scrapes, cuts, bruises, or other mild owies.

3. If there is blood present, cover with an adhesive bandage.

Benefits:

Lavender and melaleuca work together synergistically to treat skin infections, which means they work better combined than they each work alone.

Lavender and frankincense essential oils relieve the pain and anxiety that accompany owies. Often children want bandages to be placed on owies that are not bleeding because they value having their wounds attended to. Using this spray helps give them the care they desire and actually makes their owies feel better.

Witch hazel is antiseptic and astringent. It also gives the spray a consistency that applies easily.

Notes and Tips:

Aloe vera juice/gel can be used in place of the witch hazel in this recipe. If making this replacement, store the spray in the refrigerator.

A carrier oil can also be used in place of the witch hazel to make it a sprayable owie-calming rub.

MOISTURIZING HAND-SANITIZING SPRAYS

Washing your hands is the best defense against microorganisms that may make you ill. However, we aren't always someplace with soap and water readily available. Hand sanitizer is a great way to keep your hands clean; however many commercial hand sanitizers can actually make you sick if you accidentally ingest them. These hand-sanitizing spray recipes are convenient and safe for babies, children, and adults. So go out, have fun, and stay healthy.

BABY'S HAND-SANITIZING SPRAY
Ingredients:
    2 tablespoons witch hazel
    2 tablespoons vegetable glycerin
    2 drops geranium essential oil
    2 drops melaleuca essential oil
    2 drops orange essential oil

Preparation:
1. Use a metal funnel to fill a 2-ounce blue or amber glass spray bottle with 2 tablespoons vegetable glycerin.
2. Add 2 drops each of geranium, melaleuca, and orange essential oils.
3. Swirl glycerin and essential oils together.
4. Add 2 tablespoons witch hazel.
5. Apply spray nozzle cap.
6. Shake well.

KID-SAFE HAND-SANITIZING SPRAY
Ingredients:
3 tablespoon witch hazel

1 tablespoon glycerin

3 drops geranium essential oil

3 drops melaleuca essential oil

3 drops orange essential oil

2 drops clove essential oil

1 drop lemongrass essential oil

Preparation:
1. Use a metal funnel to fill a 2-ounce blue or amber glass spray bottle with 1 tablespoon vegetable glycerin.
2. Add 3 drops each of geranium, melaleuca, and orange essential oils, 2 drops clove essential oil, and 1 drop lemongrass essential oil.
3. Swirl glycerin and essential oils together.
4. Add 3 tablespoons witch hazel.
5. Apply spray nozzle cap.
6. Shake well.

Administration (for both sprays):
1. Wipe off any visible dirt from your hands.
2. Shake bottle before use.
3. Spritz a spray of the hand sanitizer in each hand.
4. Rub hands together vigorously.

Benefits:
Geranium, orange, and clove essential oils are effective against many microbes including, but not limited to *Proteus vulgaris, Pseudomonas*

aeruginosa, Escherichia coli, Staphylococcus aureus, Bacillus subtilis,
and *Klebsiella pneumoniae.*

Melaleuca has been used by Aborigines in Australia and New Zealand for its medicinal properties, for generations. Its antimicrobial properties make it superb for hand sanitation.

There are a wide variety of microbes deterred by lemongrass essential oil bacteria, but it is particularly effective against phages and fungi.

The witch hazel works as an astringent and cleanser, while the glycerin is a moisturizing carrier for the essential oils.

Notes and Tips:

The Baby's Hand-Sanitizing Spray is intended for babies ages six months to two years.

The Kid-Safe Hand-Sanitizing Spray is intended for children and adults ages two and up.

The sprays may also be used to sanitize other areas of the body, but avoid sensitive areas like the face and genitals.

If the spray gets in the eyes, rinse with carrier oil such as coconut, almond, or olive oils.

Some people have skin sensitivities to melaleuca. If the melaleuca irritates you or your child, replace it with lemon essential oil.

CHILDREN'S CHEST CONGESTION RUB

Runny noses and coughs are a common part of childhood, but that doesn't make them pleasant. Chest congestion results when the lungs are irritated and trying to expel foreign invaders such as allergens, viruses, and bacteria. Excessive coughing in turn further irritates the lungs, causing a cycle of congestion. The Children's Chest Congestion Rub soothes the lungs and supports them as they fight off viruses and bacteria.

Ingredients:

3 tablespoons coconut oil
1 tablespoon cocoa butter
2 teaspoons beeswax
6 drops lavender essential oil
4 drops cypress essential oil

2 drops cedarwood essential oil

2 drops melaleuca essential oil

Preparation:

1. Create a double boiler by putting a small glass bowl into a saucepan 1 inch full of water.
2. Over medium heat, bring the water to a simmer.
3. Melt 3 tablespoons coconut oil and 1 tablespoon cocoa butter in the glass bowl.
4. Once melted, add 2 teaspoons beeswax and heat until melted.
5. Remove glass from heat and allow mixture to cool for 4–6 minutes (making sure it's still liquified).
6. Add 6 drops lavender, 4 drops cypress, 2 drops cedarwood, and 2 drops melaleuca essential oils and stir.
7. Pour Children's Chest Congestion Rub into a metal or glass container and allow to cool.
8. Cap with an airtight lid.

Administration:

1. Rub Children's Chest Congestion Rub onto your child's chest.
2. Rub Children's Chest Congestion Rub on the bottoms of your child's feet, paying extra attention to the area next to the ball of the foot and to the top of the foot, beneath the toes.
3. Apply socks.

Benefits:

The reflexology points for the lungs and bronchial tubes exist in the area of the foot beneath the second toe down to where the arch begins and below the toes on the top of the feet.

Lavender essential oil calms sick children and soothes their lungs. It has antimicrobial properties to address infectious causes of lung congestion. Lavender essential oil helps with allergic causes of chest congestion, as well.

The antiseptic properties of melaleuca essential oils give additional support to the lungs as they fight off infections.

Cypress essential oil is stimulating to the circulation system. Healthy circulation is an important part of lung function. Cypress essential oil also acts as a nasal decongestant, which prevents postnasal drip from turning into lung congestion. Cypress's antibacterial properties address potential bacterial causes of chest congestion.

Cedarwood essential oil works as an expectorant, loosening mucus from the lungs. This allows the mucus to be expelled through productive coughs.

Notes and Tips:

The Children's Chest Congestion Rub is safe for children six months and older. For children between three and six months, dilute 1 drop lavender essential oil with 2–3 teaspoons of coconut oil and follow the administration instructions for this recipe.

If stored in a cool, dry place with a tight-fitting lid, this recipe can be stored and maintain efficacy for up to a year.

EARACHE RELIEF PROTOCOL

Earaches are a common childhood ailment. In fact, they are one of the leading cause of doctor's visits for young children. Otitis media, middle ear infection, accounts for most of these earaches. Earaches often resolve on their own with time, but the time spent waiting for the body to heal itself can be painful. This protocol soothes and relieves ear pain associated with ear infections.

Ingredients:

1–2 cotton balls
1 teaspoon coconut oil (or other carrier oil)
1 drop lavender essential oil
1 drop melaleuca essential oil (age six months and older)
1 drop basil essential oil (age two and older)

Preparation:

1. In a small glass bowl or ramekin, pour 1 teaspoon coconut oil (or other carrier oil).
2. Add 1 drop of lavender essential oil.
3. If your child is six months old or older, add 1 drop melaleuca essential oil.

4. If your child is two years old or older, add 1 drop of basil essential oil (in addition to the lavender and melaleuca essential oils).
5. Swirl to stir.
6. Soak the mixture up with a cotton ball (or two cotton balls if both ears are aching).
7. Administer immediately.

Administration:
1. Place the cotton ball(s) gently against the ear. DO NOT press into the ear canal!
2. Hold in place with your hand or with a loose cotton headband until pain subsides.
3. Wipe cotton ball behind the ear along the mastoid bone for sustained relief.

Benefits:
Lavender essential oil is analgesic, which reduces the pain of an ear infection, anti-inflammatory, which soothes the inflammation caused by infection, and antibacterial, which targets the cause of the ear infection.

Many of the bacteria and yeast that cause ear infections are susceptible to melaleuca essential oil. Melaleuca's anti-inflammatory properties calm sensitive ears.

Basil essential oil is effective against middle ear infections caused by pneumococci and *Haemophilus influenzae*.

Notes and Tips:
BE CAREFUL! Do not put essential oils directly into the ear canal.

If your child will not let you place the cotton ball against his/her ear, simply wipe the cotton ball along the mastoid bone, behind the ear.

Dogs and Cats

DOG FLEA SPRAY

Fleas love dogs, but they don't love essential oils. Essential oils are part of a plant's natural pest repellant, and you can harness this capability to rid your dog of fleas and other pests. Dogs pick up fleas easily because they need to spend time outside, but that doesn't mean you want them to bring those fleas in with them. Use the Dog Flea Spray regularly to prevent fleas from congregating on your dog and to get rid of fleas that may have already made your dog their home.

Ingredients:
1 ½ cups distilled water
¼ cup raw apple cider vinegar
2 teaspoons unscented liquid Castile soap
1 drop cedarwood essential oil
1 drop juniper berry essential oil
1 drop lavender essential oil
1 drop lemongrass essential oil

Preparation:
1. Use a funnel to pour 1 ½ cups distilled water into a 16-ounce blue or amber spray bottle.
2. Use the funnel to add ¼ cup raw apple cider vinegar and 2 teaspoons unscented liquid Castile soap.
3. Add 1 drop each cedarwood, juniper berry, lavender, and lemongrass essential oils.
4. Apply a spray nozzle top.
5. Shake to combine ingredients.

Administration:
1. Shake before use.
2. Spray the Dog Flea Spray on your dog, focusing on the areas where fleas congregate, including the neck and base of the tail.

3. Rub the spray into your dog's fur.
4. Allow to set for 5–15 minutes.
5. Rinse your dog to remove dead fleas or other insects.

Benefits:

Apple cider vinegar kills and deters fleas that are already on your dog.

Terpenoids, which can be found in a variety of essential oils, are natural and diverse pesticides. Pinene is a terpenoid found in juniper and lavender essential oils.

The pesticidal components of lemongrass essential oil include geraniol, citronellol, linalool, and limonene. Lavender essential oil also includes geraniol, linalool, and limonene.

Cedarwood essential oil protects your dog from ticks and other parasitic arthropods.

Lavender essential oil soothes your dog's skin where fleas have bitten.

Notes and Tips:

Use this spray to clean your dog's bedding and other areas where your dog frequents, like couches and carpets.

Spray a small amount of the flea spray in an area near your dog; if your dog is repulsed by the smell, do not use on your dog.

Do not let your dog lick off the Dog Flea Spray before you rinse it off.

PET-SAFE WOUND SPRAY

Just like people, pets can get bumps and scrapes from playing around or fighting. Pets are more sensitive to essential oils than humans and are also more likely to lick their wounds. Therefore, it is important to only use the mildest and safest essential oils on them for wound treatment. This Pet-Safe Wound Spray is gentle and mild, but will make your pet feel better and reduce the risk of infection.

Ingredients:

¼ cup avocado oil
8 drops lavender essential oil
4 drops Roman chamomile essential oil
1 drop bergamot essential oil (dogs only)

Preparation:

1. Use a funnel to pour ¼ cup avocado oil into a 2-ounce blue or amber glass spray bottle.
2. Add 8 drops lavender and 4 drops Roman chamomile essential oils.
3. (Optional: for dogs only) Add one drop bergamot essential oil.
4. Cap with spray cap.
5. Shake well.

Administration:

1. Allow your pet to smell the Pet-Safe Wound Spray before administering.
2. Shake well before using.
3. Spray around the wound first to see how your pet reacts.
4. Spray onto the wound.
5. If your pet will allow you, rub the spray in around the wound.

Benefits:

Lavender is antimicrobial, yet gentle.

Roman chamomile and lavender are analgesic (reducing pain), calming, anti-inflammatory, and antioxidant.

Bergamot essential oil cleanses the skin.

Avocado oil is moisturizing and contains antioxidants.

Notes and Tips:

CAUTION: Citrus oils are toxic to cats. DO NOT use the bergamot oil if you intend to use this spray with a cat.

Allow your pet to smell the spray before using it. If your pet is deterred by the aroma, do not use the wound treatment on your animal.

Spot test this recipe on your pet before using it on a wound to be sure that there is not an adverse reaction.

Adding a couple of drops of helichrysum essential oil to this recipe helps to reduce bleeding and promote healing.

Do not use this recipe in deep wounds. Instead, take your pet to the vet for stitches before using this recipe.

CAT REPELLENT SPRAY

For many people cats are wonderful companions, while others consider them a nuisance. Even if your cat is a well-loved member of your family, there may be places in your home you would like to keep cat free. For example, when cats defecate or urinate in gardens or children's play areas, it can be dangerous for your family's health. Cats cannot read signs, so keeping them where you want them can be a difficult job. This cat repellent spray not only keeps cats out of the areas you do not want them visiting, but also keeps those areas disinfected.

Ingredients:

1 cup water
½ cup vinegar
10 drops lemon essential oil
10 drops eucalyptus essential oil
5 drops rosemary essential oil
5 drops black pepper essential oil
2 drops cinnamon essential oil

Preparation:

1. Use a metal funnel to combine all ingredients in a 16-ounce blue or amber glass spray bottle.
2. Shake to combine.

Administration:

1. Spray this mixture lightly around areas you want to keep cat free.

Benefits:

Cinnamon and black pepper are irritating to cats' respiratory systems and they will avoid being around them. These oils, in addition to rosemary, help keep away other pests as well.

Lemon and eucalyptus essential oil aromas are unpleasant to cats, and this helps keep cats at bay.

The vinegar, lemon essential oil, and cinnamon essential oil are all disinfecting, so they keep the areas where you spray this mixture clean. This can be especially helpful if cats have been previously visiting those places.

Notes and Tips:

Be sure to use this spray in a well-ventilated area when cats are not around and NEVER spray this directly on cats. The limonene in the lemon essential oil cannot be processed by cats' livers and can be toxic to cats if they consume it.

If you plan to spray this on any type of fabric, make sure to test it in a small, inconspicuous spot first to be sure that it does not damage the fabric.

Do not spray this directly on your plants, but instead spray it in the dirt or around your gardens.

Spray the mixture again after rain or watering the area and on a regular basis (at least once a week).

PART THREE

Essential Oils for Natural Beauty and Spa

Self-Care with a Feminine Twist

PEPPERMINT-BERGAMOT MORNING BODYWASH

Getting up in the morning can be a daunting task. We drag ourselves out of bed and into the shower with the hope that it will wake us up enough to get us out the door. Sometimes, we even need a cup of coffee before we can make it into the shower. Peppermint essential oil, however, can be just as stimulating as a cup of coffee, and using this morning bodywash stimulates both your mind and body. Combined with peppermint, bergamot uplifts you and puts the pep in your step you need to take on a busy day.

Ingredients:
1 cup unscented liquid Castile soap
¼ cup vegetable glycerin
6 drops peppermint essential oil
6 drops bergamot essential oil

Preparation:
1. Pour a ¼ cup vegetable glycerin into a small glass bowl.
2. Add 6 drops peppermint essential oil and 6 drops bergamot essential oil.
3. Mix with a metal spoon.
4. Pour this mixture into a 16-ounce blue or amber glass bottle using a metal funnel.
5. Pour 1 cup unscented liquid Castile soap into the glass bottle using the metal funnel.
6. Cap the bottle with a pump top.
7. Shake to mix.

Administration:

1. Shake before each use—the ingredients will naturally separate between uses.
2. Pump 2–3 pumps of the morning bodywash onto a wet washcloth.
3. Rub the bodywash-covered washcloth over your skin.
4. Apply more bodywash as needed.
5. Inhale the stimulating aroma of the bodywash.
6. Rinse your entire body.

Benefits:

Peppermint essential oil stimulates your mind, increasing your cognitive functioning, and wakes you up, getting you ready for a full day, no matter how big (or small) the plans.

Bergamot essential oil relieves workplace stress and anxiety, centering you for the day ahead.

Unscented Castile soap is gentle on your skin and makes an ideal neutral base for essential oils.

Glycerin, an emulsifier, helps hold the essential oils in the mixture without the risk of rancidity that results when a carrier oil mixes with water.

The shower acts as both a humidifier and a diffuser, allowing the essential oils to work aromatically as well as topically.

Notes and Tips:

While bergamot essential oil can be phototoxic on the skin (causing sun sensitivities), this bodywash does not carry that risk because it rinses off. This is primarily a concern when the oil stays on the skin—so be sure to rinse thoroughly!

The combination of orange essential oil with peppermint essential oil is pleasant and stimulating to many people. You can substitute orange essential oil for the bergamot if you aren't seeking anxiety-relieving benefits. Orange essential oil can also be mood enhancing.

Peppermint has a cooling effect on the skin. This bodywash is perfect for a midday rinse on a hot day.

CAUTION: Be sensitive of washing your sensitive areas with this bodywash.

If you use this bodywash with a plastic pouf, you may find it does not last as long. This is because the essential oils can break down the plastic.

Washcloths are more hygienic (as long as you change them regularly) and are gentler on your skin.

EVENING FLOWER BODYWASH

A long day can leave you exhausted in mind and body, yet unable to sleep because you need time to wind down before bed while the day's events run through your mind. A soothing, warm bath or shower with this evening bodywash is a lovely solution for a busy mind and tired body. The warm water relaxes your muscles, while the scents of ylang-ylang and chamomile melt away your stresses, all preparing you for sleep.

Ingredients:
1 cup unscented liquid Castile soap
¼ cup vegetable glycerin
8 drops ylang-ylang essential oil
4 drops Roman chamomile essential oil

Preparation:
1. Pour a ¼ cup vegetable glycerin into a small glass bowl.
2. Add 8 drops ylang-ylang essential oil and 4 drops Roman chamomile essential oil.
3. Mix with a metal spoon.
4. Pour this mixture into a 16-ounce blue or amber glass bottle using a metal funnel.
5. Pour 1 cup unscented liquid Castile soap into the glass bottle using the metal funnel.
6. Cap the bottle with a pump top.
7. Shake to mix.

Administration:
1. Shake before each use—the ingredients will naturally separate between uses.
2. Pump 2–3 pumps of the evening bodywash onto a wet washcloth.
3. Rub the bodywash-covered washcloth over your skin.

4. Apply more bodywash as needed.
5. Inhale the relaxing aroma of the bodywash.
6. Rinse your entire body.

Benefits:

Ylang-ylang is a feminine, floral essential oil that calms, and decreases
   alertness.

Roman chamomile has sedative properties that soothe skin and promote
   relaxation.

Both ylang-ylang and Roman chamomile can help prevent insomnia.

Unscented Castile soap is gentle on skin and makes an ideal neutral soap
   base with essential oils.

Glycerin, an emulsifier, helps hold the essential oils in the mixture without
   the risk of rancidity that results when a carrier oil mixes with water.

The shower acts as both a humidifier and a diffuser, allowing the essential
   oils to work aromatically as well as topically.

Notes and Tips:

Use care when using this bodywash if you are co-sleeping with a young child.
The sedative effects are unlikely to be strong enough to affect your ability to
wake, but any type of sedative is not advised while co-sleeping.

If you use this bodywash with a plastic pouf, you may find the pouf does
not last as long since essential oils can break down plastic. Washcloths are
not only more durable, but they can also be more hygienic (as long they're
changed regularly) and gentler on skin.

The Relaxing Shaving Cream pairs perfectly with this bodywash.

SERENE SHAVING CREAM

Shaving your legs is a chore for some women and a time of respite for others.
The calming effects of ylang-ylang and the soft, creamy feeling of shea butter
in this recipe turn shaving time into a time of self-connection and relaxation.
Rub up your legs with this shaving cream, take some long deep breaths, take
your time with each stroke of the razor, and enjoy the transformation of your
legs from scratchy stubble to smooth, silky skin.

Ingredients:

Shaving cream base:

⅓ cup shea butter

1 tablespoon raw or Manuka honey

⅓ cup sweet almond oil

2 tablespoons unscented liquid castile soap

Essential oils:

15 drops ylang-ylang essential oil

Preparation:

1. Create a double boiler using a sauté pan and a medium glass bowl or large glass measuring cup. Fill the pan with ½-1 inch of water and bring to a soft boil on low-medium heat. Place the glass bowl/measuring cup into the water.
2. Melt ⅓ cup shea butter in the glass bowl/measuring cup.
3. Add 1 tablespoon honey and let it melt into the shea butter.
4. Remove from heat and mix in ⅓ cup sweet almond oil.
5. Place bowl in refrigerator and let contents solidify. This takes about 30 minutes to an hour.
6. Remove from refrigerator and use a hand mixer to whip the mixture until soft peaks form. Use a spatula to scrape the sides of the bowl to ensure that none of the mixture sticks to the sides.
7. Add 2 tablespoons unscented liquid castile soap and whip until fully incorporated into the mixture. This completes the shaving cream base.
8. Add 15 drops of ylang-ylang essential oil to the shaving cream base and whip for 20–30 seconds.
9. Use a metal spoon or spatula to transfer the shaving cream into one 8-ounce mason jar or two 4-ounce mason jars.
10. Apply the lid(s) and label.
11. Store away from heat and moisture.

Administration:

1. When preparing for your bath or shower, use a metal spoon to scoop two spoonfuls of the shaving cream into a small metal, glass, or ceramic bowl.
2. Fill a cup with warm water.
3. Place the bowl and glass outside of the shower or bath until you are ready to begin shaving, at which time bring both into the shower or

bathtub with you, but keep the shaving cream out of the direct stream of water.

4. Once you are ready to start shaving, take a small amount of the shaving cream and lather up the area you intend to shave.
5. Shave that area with a sharp, clean razor.
6. Rinse your blade vigorously in the cup of warm water.
7. Repeat steps 4–6 until the areas you intend to shave are completely smooth.
8. Rub the excess shower cream into the shaved areas to further moisturize and then rinse.
9. Make sure to fully wash out your razor and place it where it can dry completely.

Benefits:

Shea butter is incredibly moisturizing and protects skin from free radicals. It heals oxidative damage that has already occurred.

Honey is a powerful antibiotic and will protect your skin from bacterial colonization. If you do receive any nicks while shaving, the honey will protect them from infection.

Almond oil is easily absorbed into the skin and will clog your razor less than other carrier oils.

When ylang-ylang essential oil is absorbed through the skin, it decreases blood pressure and is exceptionally relaxing.

Notes and Tips:

The amount of ylang-ylang essential oil can be adjusted to your preference, ranging from 10–20 drops.

Shea butter is thick and does clog your razor. Makes sure to tap out the razor to remove hair and shea butter buildup and to rinse it in the cup of water regularly.

CITRUS CREAM DEODORANT

One of the best parts of aromatherapy—besides the health benefits—are the lovely smells of essential oils. Utilizing these aromas to keep ourselves smelling inviting is one of the benefits of incorporating essential oils into deodorant. Essential oils don't just mask unpleasant body odors, though—they deal with the cause of this odor. Our underarms are an excellent home for many different types of bacteria. While these bacteria may not be harmful, when they combine with sweat, they can be unpleasant to our senses. The essential oils in this recipe are antibacterial and mood lifting.

Ingredients:
⅓ cup baking soda
2–4 tablespoons almond oil
2 drops bergamot essential oil
2 drops lemon essential oil
2 drops lime essential oil
2 drops orange essential oil
1 drop melaleuca essential oil
vanilla extract (optional)

Preparation:
1. Pour ⅓ cup baking soda into a 4-ounce mason jar.
2. Start by adding 1 tablespoon almond oil and using a metal fork to stir in the oil.
3. Continue to mix in almond oil, a teaspoon at a time, until the baking soda is no longer powder. The consistency should be smooth without being oily. The amount of almond oil needed will depend on the where you live due to variations in the moisture content of the air.
4. Add 2 drops each of bergamot, lemon, lime, and orange essential oil, stirring between each oil.
5. Stir in 1 drop of melaleuca essential oil.
6. If desired, stir in vanilla extract, one drop at a time, until desired scent is achieved.
7. If needed, stir in more almond oil.
8. Use your index finger to pat down mixture down into the mason jar.
9. Seal with mason jar lid.

Administration:
1. Use your index finger to scoop out a dime-size amount of deodorant.

2. Rub the deodorant into one armpit, making sure to cover the entire armpit area.
3. Repeat on the other armpit.
4. Make sure to replace the lid tightly after using so the essential oils do not evaporate.

Benefits:

Sweating is an important part of the body's detoxification process, which is why this recipe does not call for ingredients that inhibit that process. While this is not specifically an antiperspirant, the baking soda in this recipe absorbs moisture.

Melaleuca essential oil's antimicrobial properties have been valued by Aborigines for generation upon generation and are an important part of aboriginal bush medicine. The knowledge of the benefits of melaleuca—commonly known as tea tree oil—was passed on to settlers in New Zealand and Australia, who in turn shared the information with the Western world.

Citrus essential oils are good for cleansing the skin due to their antimicrobial properties.

Citrus essential oils are incredibly uplifting. Each citrus oil in this recipe has been researched for its mood-lifting properties. Using this deodorant in the morning gives you a mood boost to get your day going.

Citrus essential oils have antioxidant properties giving this recipe additional health benefits.

Notes and Tips:

Each person has a particular scent that blends best with their body chemistry. The amounts of the individual citrus essential oil can be adjusted—while maintaining the same overall number of drops—to create a recipe that works best with your body chemistry. Grapefruit oil may be substituted for any of the citrus oils to help achieve this balance.

If you find skin sensitivity with this recipe, reduce the amount of citrus essential oils to one drop each and increase the amount of almond oil used. Discontinue use if sensitivity persists.

Much of the skin sensitivity associated with citrus oils is due to their reaction with the sun. The underarm area is rarely exposed to the sun, which makes this less of an issue with this recipe. When going out in the sun for long periods or during peak sun times, make sure to apply sunscreen to your underarms.

Man Care

WAKE-UP BODY WASH

A full day of work or school demands a keenly sharpened mind, prepared from the moment you leave the house. The first step in confronting what the world sends your way is an invigorating shower. You rouse the moment the cool water hits your body; adding the fresh scents of peppermint and rosemary to your shower stimulates the mind and body even more. Use this wake-up wash for the mental clarity and cognitive functioning you need to conquer your day.

Ingredients:
1 cup unscented liquid Castile soap
¼ cup vegetable glycerin
8 drops peppermint essential oil
4 drops rosemary essential oil

Preparation:
1. Pour a ¼ cup vegetable glycerin into a small glass bowl.
2. Add 8 drops peppermint essential oil and 4 drops rosemary essential oil.
3. Mix with a metal spoon.
4. Pour this mixture into a 16-ounce blue or amber glass bottle using a metal funnel.
5. Pour 1 cup unscented liquid Castile soap into the glass bottle, using the metal funnel.
6. Cap the bottle with a pump top.
7. Shake to mix.

Administration:
1. Shake before each use—the ingredients will naturally separate between uses.

2. Pump 2–3 pumps of the wake-up bodywash onto a wet washcloth.
3. Rub the bodywash-covered washcloth over your skin.
4. Apply more bodywash as needed.
5. Inhale the stimulating aroma of the bodywash.
6. Rinse your entire body.

Benefits:

Peppermint essential oil stimulates your mind and increases your cognitive functioning. This allows you to work at your peak ability.

Rosemary essential oil improves memory and mood. Not only will you think better at work, you'll be happier about being there.

Unscented Castile soap is gentle on your skin and is not filled with the harsh additives that many commercial washes include.

Glycerin helps hold the essential oils in the mixture without the risk of spoilage that a carrier oil carries when mixed with water.

The shower acts as a humidifier and diffuser, allowing the essential oils to work aromatically as well as topically.

Notes and Tips:

Peppermint has a cooling effect on the skin. This bodywash is perfect for a midday rinse on a hot day.

CAUTION: Be sensitive of washing your sensitive areas with this bodywash.

RESTFUL BODY WASH

A good night's sleep is often hard to get. It's easy to stay up too late, falling asleep only because your body finally crashed. Illuminated screens and other blue lights fill our days and nights, first stimulating our eyes and brains to the point of exhaustion, then interfering with our sleep cycles. With all the demands life makes, it's often difficult to set aside time to relax each night, letting the mind prepare for sleep. This restful wash helps make a bedtime shower that soothing opportunity. The sedative effects of vetiver and frankincense relax both body and mind. Follow your shower with a good book (not on a digital device), then let a good night's sleep descend upon you.

Ingredients:

1 cup unscented liquid Castile soap

¼ cup vegetable glycerin

8 drops vetiver essential oil

4 drops frankincense essential oil

Preparation:

1. Pour a ¼ cup vegetable glycerin into a small glass bowl.
2. Add 8 drops vetiver essential oil and 4 drops frankincense essential oil.
3. Mix with a metal spoon.
4. Pour this mixture into a 16-ounce blue or amber glass bottle, using a metal funnel.
5. Pour 1 cup unscented liquid Castile soap into the glass bottle, using the metal funnel.
6. Cap the bottle with a pump top.
7. Shake to mix.

Administration:

1. Shake before each use—the ingredients will naturally separate between uses.
2. Pump 2–3 pumps of the morning bodywash onto a wet washcloth.
3. Rub the bodywash-covered washcloth over your skin.
4. Apply more bodywash as needed.
5. Inhale the relaxing aroma of the bodywash.
6. Rinse your entire body.

Benefits:

Vetiver essential oil can reduce anxiety and stress, acts as a sedative, well-suited to helping you sleep. Its antioxidant properties benefit skin as well.

Frankincense is an anti-inflammatory and sedative essential oil, meaning it can calm the entire body, soothing sore muscles while preparing you for sleep. As an added benefit, it also has anticarcinogenic properties. While that does not necessarily affect its inclusion in a bodywash, this knowledge may help you sleep just a little better at night.

Unscented Castile soap is gentle on your skin and makes an ideal neutral base for soaps with essential oils.

Glycerin, an emulsifier, helps hold the essential oils in the mixture without the risk of rancidity that results when a carrier oil mixes with water.

The shower acts as both a humidifier and a diffuser, allowing the essential oils to work aromatically as well as topically.

Notes and Tips:

Vetiver is a very thick essential oil. Be patient when waiting for the drops to come out of the bottle. If the orifice reducer on your bottle becomes clogged, use a toothpick to unclog it. Do not try to rinse it clean with water.

WARM AND WOODY SHAVING CREAM

Shaving your face is a bit of an art form, requiring a steady, agile hand and the right tools. Those tools not only include the right razor, but also the right shaving cream. The Warm and Woody Shaving Cream is the shaving cream you need to achieve a close, smooth shave. It's moisturizing, healing, and will leave you feeling like a million bucks.

Ingredients:

Shaving cream base:
⅓ cup shea butter
1 tablespoon raw or Manuka honey
⅓ cup sweet almond oil
2 tablespoons unscented liquid Castile soap (optional)
Essential oils:
15 drops sandalwood essential oil

Preparation:

1. Create a double boiler using a sauté pan and a medium glass bowl or large glass measuring cup. Fill the pan with ½-1 inch of water and bring to a soft boil on low-medium heat. Place the glass bowl/ measuring cup into the water.
2. Melt ⅓ cup shea butter in the glass bowl/measuring cup.
3. Add 1 tablespoon honey and let it melt into the shea butter.
4. Remove from heat and mix in ⅓ cup sweet almond oil.

5. Place bowl in refrigerator and let contents solidify. This takes about 30 minutes to an hour.
6. Remove from refrigerator and use a hand mixer to whip the mixture until soft peaks form. Use a spatula to scrape the sides of the bowl to ensure that none of the mixture sticks to the sides.
7. (Optional) Add 2 tablespoons unscented liquid Castile soap and whip until fully incorporated into the mixture.
8. Add 15 drops of sandalwood essential oil to the shaving cream base and whip for 20–30 seconds.
9. Use a metal spoon or spatula to transfer the shaving cream into one 8-ounce mason jar or two 4-ounce mason jars.
10. Apply the lid(s) and label.
11. Store away from heat and moisture.

Administration:

How you use this shaving cream greatly depends on how you normally shave and what type of razor you use. The best shave with this shaving cream will be reached by using a safety razor or a straight razor instead of the typical disposable razor. The instructions below are for a safety razor or a typical disposable razor.

1. When preparing for your shower or sink shave, use a metal spoon to scoop one spoonful of the shaving cream into a small metal, glass, or ceramic bowl.
2. Fill a cup with warm water.
3. If showering, place the bowl and glass outside of the shower until you are ready to begin shaving at, which time bring both into the shower or bathtub with you, but keep the shaving cream out of the direct stream of water.
4. Once you are ready to start shaving, take a small amount of the shaving cream and lather up your face.
5. Allow the shaving cream to stay on your face for about one minute before beginning to shave in order to soften the hairs and moisturize the skin. Use this time to enjoy the shaving cream's mood lifting aroma.
6. Shave that area with your sharp, clean razor.
7. Rinse your blade vigorously in the cup of warm water.
8. Repeat steps 4–6 until your face is completely smooth.

9. Rub the excess shower cream into the shaved areas to further moisturize, and then rinse.
10. Make sure to fully wash out your razor and place it where it can dry completely.

Benefits:

Shea butter is incredibly moisturizing and protects skin from free radicals. It heals oxidative damage that has already occurred.

Honey is a powerful antibiotic and will protect your skin from bacterial colonization. If you do receive any nicks while shaving, the honey will protect them from infection.

Almond oil is easily absorbed into the skin.

Sandalwood essential oil acts as an astringent for your skin, while at the same time soothing your face with its cooling, antioxidant, and antispasmodic properties.

Sandalwood essential oil also increases attentiveness and mood, which brings a feeling of zen to your shaving routine.

The santalol and santyl acetate in the sandalwood essential oil are both antimicrobial, protecting your skin in case of abrasion.

Notes and Tips:

Follow with Bay Rum Aftershave to complete your shaving routine.

The amount of sandalwood essential oil can be adjusted to meet your aromatic preferences. A range of 10–20 drops of essential oil is recommended.

Shea butter is thick and does clog your razor. Makes sure to tap out the razor to remove hair and shea butter buildup and to rinse it in the cup of water regularly.

BAY RUM AFTERSHAVE

One of the manliest smells, that makes many a woman swoon, is the smell of good old-fashioned aftershave. Aftershave is an important part of the shaving routine, as it tightens the skin of the face, preventing bleeding. Beyond just its functional qualities, a good aftershave also acts as a precursor to your cologne. West Indian bay essential oil, also known as bay rum oil, began being used in the sixteenth century by European sailors who distilled *pimenta racemosa* leaves in Jamaican rum to use as a cologne. Since that time, bay rum has been associated with masculinity.

Ingredients:
4 tablespoons witch hazel
2 tablespoons dark Jamaican rum
2 teaspoons glycerin
5 drops West Indian bay essential oil
3 drops cinnamon essential oil
3 drops orange essential oil
2 drops clove essential oil

Preparation:
1. Pour 2 teaspoons glycerin into a small glass bowl.
2. Add 5 drops bay rum, 3 drops cinnamon, 3 drops orange, and 2 drops clove essential oils.
3. Whisk together glycerin and essential oils.
4. Add 4 tablespoons witch hazel and 2 tablespoons dark Jamaican rum.
5. Whisk mixture.
6. Use a metal funnel to pour into a 2-ounce blue or amber glass spray bottle.
7. Add spray top.
8. Shake vigorously.

Administration:
1. Shake before using.
2. Spray a few spritzes into your hands.
3. Rub your hands together and then pat them on your face.

Benefits:
Bay Rum essential oil is a tonic, toning the skin on the face.
Clove and cinnamon essential oils are antimicrobial, in case you have any knicks from shaving.
Clove essential oil is an analgesic, causing any of those knicks you might have not to hurt.
Orange essential oil is uplifting to the mind and body.

Witch hazel and rum are astringents, which tighten the skin and reduce bleeding from minor abrasions.

Notes and Tips:

Orange essential oil causes less photosensitivity than lemon, lime, and bergamot essential oils, but still carries some risk. Make sure to keep an eye out for any reactions to the sun. If a reaction occurs, replace with grapefruit essential oil or exclude citrus oils from the recipe.

Adding ½ teaspoon of alum powder increases the astringent properties of this recipe.

BEARD OIL

A beard says a lot about a man—the design, the length, and even the thickness. Beards, like the rest of you, need to be groomed. Beard grooming includes keeping it clean and trimmed as desired, but also using beard oil. Beard oil keeps the beard hairs soft and supple. This beard oils even helps your beard grow nice and strong.

Ingredients:

1 tablespoon jojoba oil
2 teaspoons argan oil
1 teaspoon sweet almond oil
7 drops frankincense essential oil
7 drops vetiver essential oil
5 drops West Indian bay essential oil
4 drops sandalwood essential oil
3 drops cedarwood essential oil
2 drops rosemary essential oil

Preparation:

1. Use a funnel to pour 1 tablespoon jojoba oil, 2 teaspoons argan oil, and 1 teaspoon sweet almond oil into a 2-ounce blue or amber glass bottle.
2. Swirl the oils together.
3. Add 7 drops each of frankincense and vetiver essential oils.
4. Swirl bottle to mix oils.

5. Add 5 drops West Indian bay, 4 drops sandalwood, 3 drops cedarwood, and 2 drops rosemary essential oils.
6. Top with a dropper cap.
7. Shake well.

Administration:
1. Shake before using.
2. Use the dropper to extract the beard oil from the bottle.
3. Put the desired amount of beard oil in the palm of your hand (the amount will depend on your beard length and thickness).
4. Rub the oil into your beard and into the skin beneath your beard.
5. Stroke your beard for good measure.

Benefits:
The jojoba bush is a drought-resistant shrub that grows in the deserts of California. The seeds produce jojoba oil, which is a waxy oil that smooths and softens beard hairs.

The argan tree grows in southwestern Morocco, and the kernels from its fruit are primarily harvested by women's cooperatives. The oil produced by these kernels has both internal and topical benefits. Argan oil is an antioxidant—helping skin repair from previous damage, including scars. Argan oil also has anti-sebum properties, clearing up oily skin and preventing breakouts beneath your beard.

Sweet almond oil is moisturizing and nourishing.

Frankincense is also an antioxidant, repairing prior scarring.

Frankincense, sandalwood, and vetiver's mood-enhancing properties adds to the relaxing process of beard grooming.

Vetiver acts as a base aroma for the beard oil. This allows the smell of the beard oil to change over the course of the day, yet retain a dominant base.

Rosemary and bay rum essential oils stimulate healthy hair growth.

Rosemary and cedarwood essential oils improve respiratory functioning.

Notes and Tips:
You can play with the exact proportions of the essential oils to find a balance that smells best with your beard.

Store the beard oil in a cool, dry location and use within 3–4 months.

This recipe can be doubled and still fit in a 2-ounce bottle. The amount you make will depend on the length of your beard and how much beard oil you use within 3 months.

WOODLAND CREAM DEODORANT

We all want to smell pleasant to others, but the bacteria under our arms has a different plan. Essential oil deodorant gives you the antibacterial benefits of essential oils, with the added perk of leaving your armpits smelling better than pleasant. The particular essential oils in the Woodland Cream Deodorant harness the power of wood and leaves to create an enticingly manly aroma that improves circulation and protects against prostate cancer.

Ingredients:
¼ cup arrowroot powder
¼ cup baking soda
3–5 tablespoons sweet almond oil (or other carrier oil)
8 drops sandalwood essential oil
6 drops West Indian bay essential oil
4 drops cypress essential oil
4 drops melaleuca essential oil

Preparation:
1. In a small bowl, mix together ¼ cup arrowroot powder and ¼ cup baking soda.
2. In 4-ounce mason jar, pour 2 tablespoons sweet almond oil.
3. Add 8 drops sandalwood, 6 drops West Indian bay, 4 drops cypress, and 4 drops melaleuca essential oil.
4. Mix in the oil mixture into the dry ingredients.
5. Continue to mix in sweet almond oil, 1 tablespoon at a time, until you reach an evenly moist, but not wet consistency.
6. Store mixture in the original mason jar.

Administration:
1. Use your index finger to scoop out a dime-size amount of deodorant.

2. Rub the deodorant into one armpit, making sure to cover the entire armpit area.
3. Repeat on the other armpit.
4. Make sure to replace the lid tightly after using so the essential oils do not evaporate.

Benefits:

Arrowroot powder and baking soda are moisture absorbing. Baking soda also absorbs odors.

Sandalwood essential oil is antibacterial and antifungal. It is uplifting—mentally and physically—while being beneficial for circulation. Sandalwood essential oil has the added benefit of being antitumoral, particularly in relation to prostate cancer and chemically induced skin cancer.

West Indian bay and melaleuca essential oils are antimicrobial with properties protecting against bacteria and fungi that may cause body odor.

Cypress essential oil has been used since the times of the Ancient Sumerians. Cypress essential oil improves circulation along with being antibacterial.

Notes and Tips:

This mixture can be placed into an empty stick deodorant container to create a stick-style deodorant, just reduce the amount of almond oil to make the recipe thicker.

This is not an antiperspirant; however, it does absorb moisture. If you are feeling particularly sweaty, reapply to reap more of the moisture-absorbing properties of the arrowroot and baking soda.

Make sure to store in a dry location with the lid on tightly so that the deodorant does not absorb moisture from the air.

If the deodorant feels too harsh, reduce the amount of baking soda and increase the amount of arrowroot powder. You can also reduce the amount of melaleuca essential oil to two drops.

General Personal Care

ALASKAN HAND SALVE

Cold, dry air leads to dry hands and so does hard work in the garden or anywhere where your hands are doing most the labor. Heavy-duty work requires a heavy duty hand salve. This hand salve is capable of soothing even the rough hands of an Alaskan fisherman.

Ingredients:
2 tablespoons avocado oil
2 chamomile tea bags
1 tablespoon beeswax
1 tablespoon shea butter
1 teaspoon pure lanolin
8 drops vetiver essential oil
4 drops myrrh essential oil
2 drops Roman chamomile essential oil

Preparation:
1. Warm 2 tablespoons of avocado oil in a small saucepan over low heat. This takes less than a minute.
2. Remove from heat.
3. Place 2 chamomile tea bags in a small (2–4 ounce) cup or bowl and pour the warm avocado oil over the tea bags.
4. Let the chamomile tea bags steep in the avocado oil for at least 20 minutes. (Do not start the next step until the tea bags have been steeping for at least 10 minutes.)
5. Fill another small saucepan with ½-1 inches of water and place a small (4–6-ounce) glass bowl in the saucepan. This creates a double boiler and reduces the number of dishes you'll need to wash later.

6. Melt 1 tablespoon of beeswax in this double boiler over low-medium heat. How long this takes depends on the ambient temperature—anywhere from 3–10 minutes.
7. Now add 1 tablespoon of shea butter and 1 teaspoon of pure lanolin to melt. Again, this takes between 3–10 minutes. Make sure there is still water surrounding the base of the glass bowl.
8. Once the beeswax, shea butter, and lanolin have melted, remove the glass bowl from the saucepan of water and swirl it to mix the melted ingredients together. (Using a spoon just causes the spoon to pick up the beeswax out of the mixture.)
9. Take the chamomile tea bags out of the avocado oil and squeeze them out into melted mixture in the glass bowl.
10. Pour any remaining avocado oil into the melted mixture and swirl the glass bowl to mix.
11. Add the 8 drops of vetiver essential oil and swirl.
12. Add the 4 drops of myrrh essential oil and swirl.
13. Add the 2 drops of Roman chamomile essential oil and swirl.
14. Pour the entire mixture into a 4-ounce glass mason jar or a 4-ounce stainless steel tin.
15. Put the lid on the jar or tin and let cool for 30 minutes in the refrigerator or on the counter 1–3 hours until hardened.

Administration:

1. Scrape a small amount of the salve out of the container and rub into your hands. A little goes a long way, so start small and then use more if you need it.

Benefits:

Vetiver essential oil is used throughout the perfume industry and has been utilized therapeutically in its native India since antiquity. Its main benefit in this recipe is for moisturizing and rejuvenating skin, but it also relieves stress and inflammation.

Myrrh is another ancient remedy with anti-inflammatory properties. The antimicrobial benefits of myrrh support the healing of cracked hands.

Both vetiver and myrrh have been noted to have insect-repelling qualities, which can be beneficial for those who spend a lot of time working with their hands outside.

Chamomile, both as an essential oil and in herbal form, soothes your hands and your mood.

Lanolin creates barrier on your skin, which prevents your skin from losing moisture and protects it from outside irritants.

Shea butter is moisturizing and has antioxidant benefits to protect your skin from free radical damage.

Beeswax is an excellent gelling agent, but it acts as a gentle anti-inflammatory agent, as well.

Notes and Tips:

CAUTION: Some people have a skin sensitivity to lanolin and beeswax. Make sure to test this salve on a patch of your skin before applying it to large areas.

This salve is not just for hands—it works great for feet, elbows, and knees, too.

This recipe can easily be doubled or tripled and given out as gifts for friends who garden, work with their hands a lot, or live in a cold environment.

The aroma of this salve is incredibly earthy. A couple drops of a woodsy or floral oil will balance out the aroma if it is not to your liking. Make sure to add additional essential oils after the other essential oils, but before letting it cool.

ECZEMA LOTION BAR

Eczema is itchy and irritating to children and adults alike. Scratching at it only makes it worse, and it's hard to convince a six-month-old to stop scratching. Luckily, this eczema lotion bar is perfect for everyone over six months of age. So instead of staring at your or your child's dry, flaky, itching skin and trying to will it to stop hurting and itching, grab one of these eczema lotion bars and kiss the itch good-bye.

Ingredients:

¼ cup beeswax

¼ cup shea butter

¼ cup evening primrose oil

1 tablespoon dried lavender (optional)

20 drops lavender essential oil

10 drops frankincense essential oil

10 drops Roman chamomile essential oil

Preparation:
1. Create a mock double boiler by placing a heat-safe glass bowl in a pan of simmering water.
2. Melt ¼ cup beeswax in the bowl.
3. Add ¼ cup shea butter to the melted beeswax and allow it to melt as well.
4. Swirl to mix together beeswax and shea butter.
5. Remove from heat.
6. Add ¼ cup evening primrose oil and stir.
7. Allow to cool, but not so much that it hardens.
8. Add 1 tablespoon dried lavender (optional).
9. Add 20 drops lavender, 10 drops frankincense, and 10 drops Roman chamomile essential oils.
10. Stir together all ingredients.
11. Pour into silicone molds and allow to dry until hardened (about 1–2 hours).
12. Once hardened, remove from molds and store in an airtight glass container.

Administration:
1. Remove lotion bar from airtight container.
2. Rub bar directly onto affected area.
3. Gently rub lotion into skin.
4. Return bar to airtight container.

Benefits:
Evening primrose oil, when used topically, has been found to reduce the severity of atopic eczema in children and adults.

Shea butter is a traditional African moisturizer with anti-inflammatory and analgesic properties. The inflammation of the skin affected by eczema is subdued by the shea butter, as is the itching eczema causes.

Lavender relieves the pain and itching caused by eczema.

Lavender, frankincense, and Roman chamomile are all anti-inflammatory and antioxidant essential oils, which help to soothe, calm, and heal eczema.

Notes and Tips:

For children three to six months old, exclude the frankincense essential oil and dried lavender, as well as halve the amount of lavender and Roman chamomile essential oils.

You can use silicone soap molds for larger lotion bars and silicone ice cube molds for smaller ones.

Pop a few small lotion bars into a baby food jar and keep them in your diaper bag for easy access on the go.

These bars are great for moisturizing any skin, not just areas affected by eczema.

COOLING SUNSCREEN

Protecting your skin from the sun requires a multifaceted approach. First, you need to block the UV rays that can damage your skin and cause skin damage. Next, you need to prevent your skin from becoming damaged if your skin is exposed to UV rays. And finally, you need to repair any damage that does manage to occur. The Cooling Sunscreen takes care of the first two steps by blocking the rays of the sun with good SPF-level oils and preventing damage with antioxidant oils. Complete process by using the After Sun Spray (page 134).

Ingredients:
¼ cup raw coconut oil
1 ounce grape-seed oil
45 drops peppermint essential oil
25 drops frankincense essential oil
20 drops basil essential oil
10 drops myrrh essential oil

Preparation:
1. In a 4-ounce blue or amber spray bottle, combine ¼ cup raw coconut oil with 1 ounce grape-seed oil.
2. Cap and shake well.
3. Uncap and add 40 drops peppermint, 25 drops frankincense, 20 drops basil, and 10 drops myrrh essential oils.
4. Recap and shake well.

Administration:

1. Shake well before use.
2. Spray Cooling Sunscreen onto exposed skin 30 minutes before sun exposure. (**CAUTION:** Avoid eyes.)
3. Rub Cooling Sunscreen into skin for an even coating and absorption.
4. Reapply every hour and after excessive sweating or water activities.

Benefits:

This sunscreen does not have any of the skin-damaging components of commercial sunscreens.

Coconut oil has an SPF level of 7.12, which when used consistently prevents UV rays from reaching the skin during over an hour of sun exposure. While this may sound low, it can provide substantial skin protecting benefits over a lifetime.

Grape seeds contain a high level of polyphenols, which act as UV blockers. Grape-seed oil is also an antioxidant, which protect skin from the damaging effects of the sun.

Peppermint essential oil has an SPF of 6.67, making it one of the most sun-protective essential oils. Peppermint essential oil is also cooling and feels refreshing when applied to hot skin.

The phenolic acid in basil essential oil is also a UV blocker, and basil essential oil has been found to have good sunscreen activity.

Myrrh and frankincense essential oils are highly antioxidative. They protect and rejuvenate skin that has exposed to the sun.

Notes and Tips:

Following sun exposure, use the After Sun Spray that comes next in this book.

This sunscreen is not waterproof and should be applied 30 minutes before sun exposure and reapplied after every hour of sun exposure and after getting wet.

CAUTION: If you get this sunscreen in your eyes, flush with grape-seed oil (or other carrier oil), not water.

CAUTION: Peppermint essential oil may react negatively on the lung function of some young children. DO NOT use peppermint essential oil with children under the age of six.

Replace the peppermint essential oil with lavender essential oil, which has an SPF of 5.62, to make this sunscreen safe for children ages 2 and above.

To increase the SPF level of this sunscreen, considering adding zinc powder.

AFTER SUN SPRAY

After sun exposure, it's important to continue the skin protection that sunscreen starts. Skin exposed to UV rays benefits from continued protection by antioxidants; those antioxidants also repair damage the the UV rays have caused. If skin has been sunburned, it needs soothing. The After Sun Spray protects, repairs, and soothes sun-exposed skin.

Ingredients:
¼ cup aloe vera juice
¼ cup aloe vera gel
2 green tea bags
15 drops Roman chamomile essential oil
15 drops frankincense essential oil
5 drops clove essential oil

Preparation:
1. In a small saucepan over medium heat, bring ¼ cup aloe vera juice to a simmer. (Watch closely as this happens quickly.)
2. Turn off heat and pour into a small teacup.
3. Steep 2 green tea bags in the aloe vera juice for 10 minutes.
4. Remove tea bags—squeezing out any excess liquid from the tea bags— and add ¼ cup of aloe vera gel.
5. Use a funnel to pour the aloe vera tea into a 4-ounce blue or amber glass spray bottle.
6. Add 15 drops each of Roman chamomile and frankincense essential oils.
7. Add 5 drops of clove essential oil.
8. Cap bottle with a spray cap and shake well.
9. Store in the refrigerator.

Administration:

1. Shake well.
2. Spray onto sun-exposed skin, immediately after sun exposure.
3. Gently rub into skin.

Benefits:

Green tea is one of the most highly antioxidant plants available. Its benefits can be used topically in addition to its traditional internal uses.

Aloe vera gel is well known for its skin care benefits, particularly in healing burns and inflamed skin.

Roman chamomile and frankincense essential oils are soothing for the skin due to their anti-inflammatory and antioxidant properties.

Clove essential oil is also highly protective against free radicals and is an antioxidant. It also works as an analgesic to numb the pain that overexposure to the sun can cause.

Notes and Tips:

This spray is safe to use with children over the age of two.

People with ragweed allergies are at an increased risk of developing skin sensitivities to chamomile. If you are allergic to ragweed, first decrease the amount of chamomile in the recipe (replace with lavender essential oil). Then, spot test the spray before using it over a large area. Do not skip this step! Additionally, be aware of your body's reaction to the spray after multiple uses. Discontinue use (and remake, completely replacing the Roman chamomile with lavender) if sensitivities arise. However, the risk of contact dermatitis is low, and a ragweed allergy doesn't mean an automatic sensitivity to chamomile essential oil.

If you only have aloe vera gel, and not aloe vera juice, you can replace the juice with the gel. However, you must heat it in a double boiler, instead of directly in a sauce pan. Also, remove the spray from the refrigerator before you go out in the sun, so that it can liquify enough before use to be sprayable.

When stored in the refrigerator, a bottle of After Sun Spray can last an entire season—up to three months.

GENTLE ROSEMARY-ORANGE SHAMPOO

Over shampooing can dry out your scalp. This in turn causes your oil glands to overcompensate for your arid scalp, produce too much oil, and cause oily hair. This cycle of dried-out and then overly oily scalp and hair can be hard to beat. However, taking a break from traditional shampoos can give your scalp a rest and a chance to get back to a more natural oil production cycle. The Gentle Rosemary-Orange Shampoo moisturizes your scalp, while gently cleansing your hair.

Ingredients:
¾ cup unscented liquid Castile soap
¾ cup canned coconut milk
3 tablespoons jojoba oil
1 teaspoon vitamin E oil
10 drops rosemary essential oil
10 drop orange essential oil

Preparation:
1. Use a funnel to combine ¾ cup unscented liquid Castile soap with ¾ cup canned coconut milk in a 16-ounce blue or amber bottle.
2. Add 3 tablespoons jojoba oil.
3. Add 1 teaspoon vitamin E oil.
4. Add 10 drops each rosemary and orange essential oil.
5. Cap with a pump top.
6. Shake to combine ingredients.

Administration:
1. Shake before using.
2. Wet your hair.
3. Pump desired amount of Gentle Rosemary-Orange Shampoo into the palm of your hand.
4. Rub shampoo into your scalp and through your hair.
5. Rinse with warm water.

Benefits:
Unscented liquid Castile soap is gentle as it cleanses your hair and scalp.
Coconut milk moisturizes and nourishes your hair.
Vitamin E oil maintains the freshness of the Gentle Shampoo because of its antioxidant properties.

Jojoba oil helps smooth hair and keep it moisturized.

Rosemary essential oil stimulates the scalp and encourages hair growth.
Rosemary prevents fungal infections from developing on the scalp.

Orange essential oil complements the aroma of the rosemary essential oil. It is also cleansing for the hair.

Notes and Tips:

Follow with the Conditioning Rinse found on page 137.

For oily hair, reduce the amount of jojoba oil to 1 tablespoon.

This shampoo will last longer if kept in the refrigerator between uses.

This recipe can also be frozen in silicone ice cube trays, and a single cube can be used per hair wash.

There is usually a transitional period where your hair gets used to a milder shampoo and may continue to overproduce oil. This period usually lasts about one week.

CONDITIONING HAIR RINSE

Conditioners are intended to smooth your hair and leave it shining, but many traditional conditioners also weigh your hair down. This conditioning hair rinse leaves your hair soft, light, and manageable. Plus, the aromas of clary sage, ylang-ylang, and sandalwood do the same thing for your mood.

Ingredients:

1 cup distilled water

2 tablespoons raw apple cider vinegar

3 drops clary sage essential oil

3 drops ylang-ylang essential oil

2 drops sandalwood essential oil

Preparation:

1. In a 12–16-ounce glass, combine 1 cup distilled water and 2 tablespoons raw apple cider vinegar.
2. Add 3 drops clary sage essential oil, 3 drops ylang-ylang essential oil, and 2 drops sandalwood essential oil.
3. Swirl to combine ingredients.

Administration:

1. After rinsing out your shampoo, pour the Conditioning Hair Rinse over your hair.
2. Use a comb to evenly distribute the rinse through your hair.
3. Leave in your hair or rinse your hair with cool water.

Benefits:

Apple cider vinegar balances the pH levels of your hair and closes the hair follicles to prevent damage to the hair. It also leaves your hair shiny.

Clary sage, ylang-ylang, and sandalwood essential oils are all promote a relaxed mood and feelings of well-being.

Clary sage essential oil helps to prevent head lice from making their home in your hair.

Sandalwood essential oil protects your scalp from skin cancer.

Ylang-ylang essential oil strengthens your hair to prevent split ends.

Notes and Tips:

Use with the Gentle Rosemary-Orange Shampoo found on page 135.

For drier hair, reduce the amount of apple cider vinegar to 1 tablespoon.

This rinse is intended to be used within an hour of preparation, but if you want to make it in advance, use a mason jar instead of a glass and cap it tightly. Store in the refrigerator for up to a week.

DANDRUFF PROTOCOL

Dandruff can come in several forms. It can be dry and flaky, or it can be oily and almost scaly. Either form can be itchy, and itching your scalp can irritate the skin, making the original problem worse. While dandruff is usually a harmless condition, it can be uncomfortable and unsightly. This dandruff protocol helps soothe and hydrate the scalp, while at the same time preventing infection and clearing away excess scalp flakes.

Ingredients:

3 tablespoons jojoba oil
4 drops melaleuca essential oil
4 drops lavender essential oil

4 drops rosemary essential oil

2 drops Roman chamomile essential oil

Preparation:

1. In a small glass or bowl, combine all ingredients.
2. Stir ingredients together with a metal spoon.

Administration:

1. Use your fingers to gently massage the mixture through your hair, directly onto your scalp. Pay special attention to the areas where the scalp is flaking.
2. Cover your hair with a cloth and let the mixture rest in your hair for at least six hours.
3. Take the cloth off your hair and massage the scalp again.
4. If there are patches of oily, scaly scalp, use a fine-toothed comb to gently remove these patches from the scalp and pull them out of your hair.
5. Wash your hair as you would normally to remove excess flakes and oils.

Benefits:

Melaleuca and rosemary essential oils both have antimicrobial properties to protect the scalp from potential infections.

Rosemary essential oil also stimulates the blood flow to the scalp, which supports general scalp health.

Lavender and Roman chamomile essential oils soothe the scalp to prevent itching.

Jojoba oil helps the scalp retain moisture and is easily absorbed by the scalp.

Notes and Tips:

Test the essential oil mixture on your arm first to make sure it does not irritate your skin. If it does, increase the amount of jojoba oil and test again. If it continues to irritate you, do not use.

This protocol can be begun at night before going to bed, so that you can sleep as it is working. When using this protocol at night, the lavender and Roman chamomile essential oils have the added benefits of supporting your sleep.

This protocol can be administered regularly to support scalp health.

ORAL HEALTH MOUTH RINSE

Oral health is about a lot more than fresh breath, but fresh breath is a pleasant benefit of a healthy mouth. Keeping your mouth clean with regular brushing and flossing is the first step to keeping your teeth clean, but your gums, upper throat, palate, and inner checks all need attention, too. The Oral Health Mouth Rinse addresses these parts along with your teeth by preventing plaque buildup, stopping gingivitis, and preventing oral cancers.

Ingredients:

1 ounce warm distilled water
1 teaspoon raw honey
1 drop basil essential oil
1 drop clove essential oil
1 drop melaleuca essential oil
1 drop eucalyptus essential oil
1 drop myrrh essential oil

Preparation:

1. Pour 1 teaspoon honey into a glass shot glass.
2. Add 1 drop each of basil, clove, and melaleuca essential oils.
3. Add 1 ounce warm distilled water.
4. Add 1 drop each of eucalyptus and myrrh essential oils.

Administration:

1. Pour the contents of the shot glass into your mouth.
2. Swish the liquid around your mouth for approximately one minute, making sure to get between your teeth, all around your gums, and your inner cheeks.
3. Gargle for about 15 seconds.
4. Spit out Oral Health Mouth Rinse.

Benefits:

Myrrh has been used for oral health since ancient times. Myrrh is beneficial for the gums and soothes inflammation in the mouth. It is particularly soothing for mouth ulcers. The antiseptic and astringent properties of myrrh keep the mouth, including teeth, gums, tongue, and throat clean.

Clove essential oil is incredibly antiseptic and cleans the mouth very well. Its analgesic properties numb any mouth or tooth pain you may be experiencing.

The combination of basil, clove, and melaleuca has been found to have antiplaque and antigingivitis properties.

Eucalyptus essential oil has been used in dentistry for many years due to its antiplaque, antibacterial, anti-inflammatory, and cancer-preventing mechanisms.

Honey is antibacterial and helps to dilute the essential oils.

Notes and tips:

You can heat the honey with the distilled water if you do not like the consistency of the honey.

If you find your lips are sensitive to the essential oils in this rinse, use a lip balm to protect them before using the mouth rinse.

Home Spa

COCONUT LIME VERBENA SUGAR SCRUB

Sugar scrubs are wonderful way to exfoliate your skin, while at the same time allowing yourself a little bit of luxury. Store-bought sugar scrubs can be surprisingly expensive, but the ingredients for a homemade sugar scrub are simple and inexpensive. This coconut lime verbena sugar scrub brings a tropical spa feel into your bathtub or shower.

Ingredients:

1 cup raw sugar

2 tablespoons raw coconut oil

10 drops lime essential oil

1 tablespoon dried lemon verbena leaves, crushed

Preparation:

1. Soften your coconut oil either in the microwave (using a glass bowl) for 10 seconds at a time or on the stove at low heat.
2. Place 1 cup of sugar in a medium-size glass bowl.
3. Add 2 tablespoons coconut oil to the mixture slowly, stirring as you pour it into the sugar.
4. Add 10 drops of lime essential oil one drop at a time, stirring between each drop.
5. Sprinkle in the dried verbena and stir to evenly distribute it through the mixture.
6. Divide the sugar scrub between two 4-ounce mason jars and put the lids on tightly.

Administration:

1. Before getting into the bath or shower, use a spoon to scoop out your desired amount of sugar scrub into a small dish.

2. After wetting your skin, use your hands to rub the sugar scrub over your arms, shoulders, stomach, back, hips, legs, and feet. Avoid your face and sensitive areas.
3. Rinse the sugar scrub off your body using warm water. As you rinse off the sugar and verbena, massage the coconut oil into your skin.

Benefits:

Raw sugar is larger and rougher than refined sugar and therefore is more exfoliating. The coconut oil protects your skin, while the raw sugar removes dead skin cells.

Lime essential oil is uplifting to the mood.

Lemon verbena leaves contain constituents with antispasmodic properties.

Notes and Tips:

Additional raw coconut oil can be added to this recipe if you prefer a more oily consistency.

Other citrus essential oils such as bergamot, lemon, or wild orange essential oils can be substituted for the lime essential oil as they have similar mood-lifting properties.

Lime essential oil contains limonene, which causes sun sensitivity when used on the skin. So while this sugar scrub smells like a tropical beach vacation, it is not recommended that it be used directly before sun exposure. The raw coconut oil does provide protection from the sun, but the protective ability of coconut oil against limonene phototoxicity has not been studied.

SWEET AND SUBTLE SUGAR SCRUB

Part of pampering yourself is giving yourself something sweet, but it doesn't always have to come in the form of food. Your skin deserves a sweet treat on those pampering days or even every day. This sugar scrub is that perfect gift to your body. It delights the senses, while being gentle on the skin.

Ingredients:

1 cup refined sugar
2 tablespoons light olive oil
4 drops ylang-ylang essential oil

2 drops geranium essential oil
2 drops sandalwood essential oil

Preparation:

1. Place 1 cup of sugar in a medium-size glass bowl.
2. Add 2 tablespoons sweet almond oil to the mixture slowly, stirring as you pour it into the sugar.
3. Add 4 drops ylang-ylang, 2 drops geranium, and 2 drops sandalwood essential oils, one drop at a time. Stir between each drop.
4. Divide the sugar scrub between two 4-ounce mason jars and put the lids on tightly.

Administration:

1. Before getting into the bath or shower, use a spoon to scoop out your desired amount of sugar scrub into a small dish.
2. After wetting your skin, use your hands to rub the sugar scrub over your arms, shoulders, stomach, back, hips, legs, and feet. Avoid your face and sensitive areas.
3. Rinse the sugar scrub off your body using warm water.

Benefits:

Refined sugar is gentler on the skin than raw sugar and is ideal for softer or more sensitive skin.

The germacrene in ylang-ylang, cintronellol in geranium, and α-santalol in sandalwood are all antioxidants. Olive oil is also an antioxidant due to its phenolic compounds.

Antioxidants reduce skin roughness and scaling.

Notes and Tips:

Light olive oil is used in this recipe due to its subtle aroma. However, any olive oil can be used, and darker olive oils do have higher antioxidant benefits.

Additional olive oil can be added to this recipe if you prefer a more oily consistency.

Make sure to rinse your shower or tub thoroughly after using any scrub to keep the floor from becoming slippery.

INVIGORATING, CELLULITE-REDUCING SALT SCRUB

Cellulite is a normal part of being a human. It affects women significantly more than men, but the presence of cellulite occurs in people of all sizes. Cellulite is not a medical condition, but it is a cosmetic one and many people would like to see a reduction in the appearance of dimpling on their thighs and buttocks. This salt scrub not only reduces the unsightly appearance of cellulite, it also helps you slim your thighs and hips.

You don't have to have cellulite to enjoy this scrub. The invigorating aspects of the scrub—coffee and grapefruit, orange, and rosemary essential oils—make this scrub a splendid way to start your morning. Plus, you still get to enjoy smoother, softer skin.

Ingredients:
¼ cup epsom salts
¼ cup ground coffee beans
3 tablespoons jojoba oil
8 drops grapefruit essential oil
5 drops orange essential oil
4 drops black pepper essential oil
3 drops rosemary essential oil
1 drop cinnamon essential oil
1 drop ginger essential oil

Preparation:
1. In a glass bowl, combine 3 tablespoons jojoba oil with 8 drops grapefruit, 5 drops orange, 4 drops black pepper, 3 drops rosemary, 1 drop cinnamon, and 1 drop ginger essential oils. Stir oils together with a metal whisk.
2. Add ¼ cup epsom salts to the oil mixture and stir until oils are evenly distributed throughout the epsom salts.
3. Add ¼ cup coffee grounds to the mixture and stir until the salt scrub is evenly mixed.
4. Place two spoonfuls of the scrub in a small glass, metal, or ceramic bowl to use immediately.

5. Store the rest of the scrub in a 4-ounce mason jar for use later or to give as a gift.

Administration:

1. Before getting into the bath or shower, use a spoon to scoop out your desired amount of Invigorating Salt Scrub into a small dish.
2. After wetting your skin, use your hands to rub the salt scrub over your arms, shoulders, stomach, back, hips, legs, and feet. Avoid your face and sensitive areas.
3. Rinse the salt scrub off your body, using warm water.

Benefits:

Caffeine is a common ingredient in cellulite creams. It reduces thigh and buttocks circumference and the dimpling appearance of cellulite. It does this by preventing the overaccumulation of fat within cells.

Jojoba oil increases the caffeine release from the coffee grounds and makes it more readily available for absorption by your skin.

Used topically, orange, black pepper, cinnamon, and ginger reduce the appearance of cellulite.

Use aromatically, grapefruit and black pepper essential oils affect the sympathetic nervous system. When combined with topical caffeine absorption, this has a slimming effect and reduces fat accumulation.

Rosemary essential oil is invigorating and stimulating to the mind.

Notes and Tips:

If kept in a cool, dark, and dry place, this scrub will last over two months and maintain its efficacy. How long it lasts will depend on the freshness of the ingredients, how infrequently it is opened and the moisture and heat levels in the air.

Even though grapefruit is a citrus oil, it does not have the phototoxicity issues that other citrus oils can have. Therefore, it is safe to use on skin that will be exposed to the sun.

The antioxidants in coffee protect skin from the effects of sun damage including early aging, skin cancer, and photosensitive erythema (a rash or redness due to oversensitivity to the sun).

Using coffee from East Africa—such as Kenyan, Ethiopian, or Tanzanian coffees—for the coffee grounds will pair well with the grapefruit and orange essential oil in this recipe. Latin American coffees will also add a pleasant citrus aroma when used in this recipe. Asian Pacific coffees will emphasize the cinnamon essential oil.

Lighter roasted coffees have a higher caffeine content than darker roasts.

ORANGE BLOSSOM HONEY SALT SCRUB

Smooth, nourished skin feels sensational. Pair that with the sweet smell of orange blossom honey, the bright aroma of orange essential oil, and fragrant geranium essential oil, and well, you've got yourself the recipe for a luxurious shower. Scrub your whole body with the Orange Blossom Honey Salt Scrub and feel the difference it makes to your skin.

Ingredients:
½ cup epsom salts
¼ cup ground Himalayan crystal salts
3 tablespoons orange blossom honey
2 tablespoons sweet almond oil
1 tablespoon evening primrose oil
10 drops orange essential oil
2 drops geranium essential oil

Preparation:
1. In a large glass bowl, whisk together 2 tablespoons sweet almond oil, 1 tablespoon evening primrose oil, and 3 tablespoons orange blossom honey.
2. Whisk in 10 drops orange and 2 drops geranium essential oils.
3. Stir in ½ cup epsom salts and ¼ cup Himalayan salts.
4. Stir until evenly mixed.
5. Divide between three 4-ounce mason jars and cap tightly.

Administration:
1. Before getting into the bath or shower, use a spoon to scoop out your desired amount of Orange Blossom Honey Salt Scrub into a small dish.
2. After wetting your skin, use your hands to rub the salt scrub over your arms, shoulders, stomach, back, hips, legs, and feet. Avoid your face and sensitive areas.
3. Rinse the salt scrub off your body using warm water.

Benefits:

Evening primrose oil contains gamma-linolenic acid, an essential fatty acid for skin health, which improves skin elasticity and smoothness.

Himalayan pink salts are nourishing to your skin, containing a variety of compounds not found in traditional table salts.

The combination of orange blossom honey and orange essential oil cleanses your skin without drying it out.

Geranium essential oil's anti-inflammatory properties are particularly effective against edema, swelling of the skin due to fluid build up.

Notes and Tips:

If you use the same tablespoon to measure the honey as you do the primrose oil, the honey will release from the tablespoon easily.

Getting water in your container of bath salts will decrease the longevity of the Orange Blossom Honey Salt Scrub due to the contamination of the almond oil putting it at risk for rancidity. Make sure to use dry hands or a spoon to scoop out the desired amount of scrub into a separate container before getting into the bath or shower.

SERENE SOAK BATH SALTS

One of the best parts of an expansive spa experience is the mineral baths. The hot—almost too hot—water, the steam rising toward your face, the slow release of tension from your muscles all ease you in to a place of pure serenity. Achieving this at home can seem like a daunting task, but this recipe gives you exactly what you need to turn your bathtub into a spa-inspired mineral bath. The experience is furthered by the aromatherapy that will be wafting up with the steam. This recipe includes an incredibly serene combination of essential oils meant to take your entire body into a state of bliss.

Ingredients:

½ cup epsom salts

¼ cup finely ground pink Himalayan crystal salt

¼ cup mineral salts

5 drops ylang-ylang essential oil

4 drops lavender essential oil

3 drops sandalwood essential oil

2 drops Roman chamomile essential oil

1 drop geranium essential oil

Preparation:

1. In a large glass bowl, combine ½ cup epsom salt and ¼ each of Himalayan and mineral salts.
2. Stir until the salts are evenly blended.
3. One drop at a time, stir in 5 drops ylang-ylang, 4 drops lavender, 3 drops sandalwood, 2 drops Roman chamomile, and 1 drop geranium essential oils.
4. Continue to stir until the essential oils have been evenly distributed among the salts.
5. Divide the salts between three 4-ounce mason jars.
6. Apply the lids tightly and label each jar.

Administration:

1. Begin drawing a bath with hot water.
2. Add 2–3 tablespoons of Serene Soak Bath Salts to your bath when it is about halfway full.
3. Get in the bath and stir the bathwater with your hands so that the salts dissolve as the tub fills to your desired depth.
4. Lay back and soak your body in the salt bathwater.

Benefits:

Ylang-ylang and lavender, both alone and combined, reduce psychological stress, blood pressure, and pulse rates.

Geranium and lavender are sedative essential oils, making this soak a superb choice for before bedtime or even a midday nap.

Sandalwood and Roman chamomile are calming for the mind and body.

Roman chamomile is renowned for its anti-inflammatory properties, allowing your joints to join in the relaxation.

Mineral salts are the essence of balneotherapy, the therapeutic use of salts and warm water.

Geranium essential oil also has anti-cancer benefits, which—while not the purpose of this soak—can give you a little extra peace of mind.

Himalayan crystal salts are mined from mountains in the Himalayas. They form in the presence of other elements and compounds beyond just sodium chloride. This adds to the variety of elements in this recipe and increases its balneotherapeutic benefits.

Notes and Tips:
Add to the ambiance of your bath by lighting candles, playing soft music, and turning off the lights.

Make sure that you do not stay too long in the tub, as you may start to get sleepy.

If stored in a cool, dark place, these bath salts can last for two years or more. Just be sure to keep the lid on tightly. The more often you open the jar, the less effective the bath salts will become due to evaporation of the essential oils.

BERGAMOT BUTTER BATH BOMBS

Even grown-ups deserve to have fun in the bath. These Bergamot Butter Bath Bombs put a twist on the bubble bath. Instead of the bubbles forming on top of the bath, the bath bombs fizz under the water, releasing the luxurious aroma of bergamot, frankincense, and cocoa butter. Your skin will be left moisturized and your senses will be tantalized.

Ingredients:
1 ½ cups baking soda
½ cup cornstarch
½ cup citric acid
2 tablespoons cocoa butter
1–2 tablespoons witch hazel (in a spray bottle)
20 drops bergamot essential oil, divided
10 drops frankincense essential oil

Preparation:
1. In a medium-size glass mixing bowl, combine 1 ½ cups baking soda with ½ cup cornstarch.

2. Mix with a metal spoon.
3. In a separate small glass bowl, melt 2 tablespoons cocoa butter in the microwave or double boiler.
4. Add 10 drops of bergamot essential oil to the melted cocoa butter.
5. Very slowly add the cocoa butter and bergamot essential oil mixture to baking soda and cornstarch mixture. Use your hands to blend the mixture between adding a few drops at a time.
6. Once the mixture is evenly combined, stir in ½ cup citric acid.
7. Spritz in witch hazel, one spritz at a time and use your hands to evenly mix in the witch hazel.

   Note: Be sure not to let the mixture get too wet or the citric acid will activate and start to bubble.

   CAUTION: If you have sensitive skin or any cuts or scrapes on your hands, use gloves when mixing in the witch hazel.
8. Once the mixture is damp enough to be malleable, scoop it into ten silicone molds of your choice, pressing down firmly as you fill the molds.
9. Apply pressure again to the top of each filled mold.
10. Allow to dry in the open air for 24 hours.
11. Remove bath bombs from molds and add 1 drop of bergamot and 1 drop of frankincense to the top of each one.
12. Store in an airtight glass container.

Administration:
1. Use dry hands to remove one Bergamot Butter Bath Bomb from the container.
2. Draw yourself a bath.
3. When you are about to get into your bath, drop in your Bergamot Butter Bath Bomb.
4. Climb in the tub and relax.

Benefits:
Cocoa butter is a traditional African moisturizer for sensitive skin.

The combination of bergamot and frankincense essential oils improves mood.

The fizz is just plain fun!

Notes and Tips:

The Bergamot Butter Bath Bombs are safe to use for children ages two and above.

Make sure the Bergamot Butter Bath Bombs are completely dry before removing them from the silicone molds and make sure to remove them carefully to prevent crumbling.

CAUTION: If you have any open cuts or scrapes, citric acid can sting.

PEDICURE PREP PROTOCOL

Whether you are planning for a day at the spa, your local nail salon, or some personal pampering at home, the perfect pedicure takes some preparation. Healthy toenails are the first step to getting your feet ready for polish or nail wraps, but this can be hampered by weak nails or nail fungus. Luckily, the Healthy Nail Oil can strengthen and heal unhealthy nails. Once your nails are in tip-top shape, it's time to get your feet smooth, fresh, and sandal ready. The Soothing Foot Soak and the Smoothing Foot Scrub combine to exfoliate and moisturize, plus both relax and stimulate tired feet. After following the Pedicure Prep Protocol, your feet will be ready to hit the beach or curl up under the covers, wherever they will be happiest, with or without nail decoration.

This protocol is meant to be conducted in the sequence that the recipes are presented. Use the Healthy Nail Oil first, followed by the Soothing Foot Soak, and finish with the Smoothing Foot Scrub. Preparing the Smoothing Foot Scrub before the Soothing Foot Soak, however, will save you the hassle of trying to prepare the scrub with wet feet, and you won't have to re-wet your feet to use the scrub.

HEALTHY NAIL OIL
Ingredients:

1 teaspoon coconut oil
1 drop melaleuca essential oil
1 drop lavender essential oil
1 drop lemon essential oil

Preparation:

1. In a glass, metal, or ceramic ramekin, mix together 1 teaspoon coconut oil with 1 drop each of melaleuca, lavender, and lemon essential oils, using a metal spoon.

Administration:

1. Apply the Healthy Nail Oil onto each nail, covering the nail fully.
2. Rub around the cuticle of each toenail.
3. Use a wooden cuticle stick to apply the oil under each toenail.
4. Let the oil set while you prepare the Smoothing Foot Scrub and Soothing Foot Soak.
5. Rinse the oil off in the Soothing Foot Soak or leave on until your next bath or shower.

SOOTHING FOOT SOAK
Ingredients:

10 cups hot water

1 cup apple cider vinegar

¼ cup epsom salts

¼ cup mineral salts

6 drops lemongrass essential oil

4 drops lavender essential oil

2 drops Roman chamomile essential oil

Preparation:

1. In a glass bowl, combine ¼ epsom salts, ¼ cup mineral salts, 6 drops lemongrass essential oil, 4 drops lavender essential oil, and 2 drops Roman chamomile. Stir ingredients together until they are evenly combined.
2. In a foot bath or large container, combine 10 cups hot water and 1 cup apple cider vinegar.
3. Add salt and essential oil mixture to the foot bath. Stir to dissolve the salts.

Administration:

1. Place your feet into the foot bath.
2. Let your feet soak for 10–20 minutes, until the water becomes tempid.
3. Immediately follow with Uplifting Foot Scrub.

SMOOTHING FOOT SCRUB
Ingredients:
- ¼ cup epsom salts
- 1 tablespoon coconut oil, liquified
- 5 drops peppermint essential oil
- 4 drops lime essential oil

Preparation:
1. In a glass bowl, combine 1 tablespoon liquid coconut oil, 5 drops peppermint, and 4 drops lime essential oil. Stir oils together with a metal or wooden spoon.
2. Add ¼ cup epsom salts to the oil mixture and stir until oils are evenly distributed throughout the epsom salts.

Administration:
1. Begin with your feet either over a towel by a sink or in the shower.
2. Use your hand to scoop approximately a quarter of the scrub from the bowl.
3. Massage the scrub into one of your wet/damp feet (your feet should still be at least damp from the Soothing Foot Soak).
4. Scoop another quarter of the scrub into your hand and massage your other foot.
5. Use the remaining scrub to exfoliate any particularly rough areas of your feet, such as your heels.
6. Rinse your feet in the sink or shower with warm water.
7. Pat your feet dry with a towel and allow them to fully air dry before putting on shoes or socks.

Benefits:
Peppermint essential oil is stimulating to the mind and helps relieve muscle pain. It is also fungistatic, inhibiting the growth fungus that may affect the feet.

Melaleuca and lavender are antifungal individually, but also work synergistically to increase their antifungal properties beyond what would be expected by just adding them together.

Roman chamomile and lavender are both antimicrobial essential oils with anti-inflammatory and sedative mood properties. They soothe and relax your feet and your mind.

Adding lavender essential oil to a foot bath affects the autonomic activity of the body, relaxing you from the outside in.

Lemongrass essential oil is one of the most powerful antifungal essential oils. The addition of heat and salt increases its antifungal abilities.

Lemon and lime essential oils are both cleansing oils with mood-enhancing properties—perfect for a spa-like experience.

Balneotherapy, the use of heated, mineral-rich water to treat disease, is an ancient practice that has become part of modern medicinal practices. The addition of the mineral salts to the foot soak helps relieve foot pain and soreness.

Epsom salt, a.k.a. magnesium sulfate, is well known as a treatment for muscle aches and pains. The size of the salt crystals makes it an excellent exfoliant.

Coconut oil is not only moisturizing to the skin, but also helps soothe sore feet with its anti-inflammatory properties. Like the essential oils used in these recipes, coconut oil has antifungal properties.

Notes and Tips:

The Healthy Nail Oil is great for the nails on your hands, too.

Using a pumice stone to scrub your feet, with the Smoothing Foot Scrub, will increase the amount of dead skin you can remove with this recipe. However, using your hands gives you silken hands—preparing you for a manicure, too!

Preparing the Smoothing Foot Scrub before the Soothing Foot Soak saves you from walking around with wet feet and from having your feet dry out before administering the scrub.

All recipes can be made into larger batches and stored for several months in airtight glass containers. The Soothing Foot Soak should be made without the vinegar or hot water for storage purposes. The premade salt and oil base can be added to the vinegar and hot water at the time of use.

BURST OF ENERGY MEDITATION DIFFUSER BLEND

Meditation can be energizing and relaxing depending on its purpose. Use the Burst of Energy Meditation Diffuser Blend when you are looking to awaken your mind, body, and spirit, while bringing them into harmony. The bright burst of citrus stimulates the left side of your brain, giving it the ingenuity to come up with innovative solutions for queries you may be pondering during your meditation. This blend is splendid for when you take a break during your hectic day or even a great way to start the morning.

Ingredients:
½ cup water
10 drops grapefruit essential oil
2 drops rosemary essential oil

Preparation:
1. Add ½ cup of water to your diffuser (or the amount recommended in your diffuser's instructions).
2. Add 10 drops grapefruit and 2 drops rosemary essential oils.

Administration:
1. Find an interruption-free place to meditate.
2. Plug in your diffuser near where you will be meditating.
3. Turn on your diffuser with the Burst of Energy Meditation Blend in it.
4. Inhale deeply as you meditate.

Benefits:
Grapefruit essential oil is uplifting to the mind, body, and spirit. It opens up the pathways to the right side of the brain, increasing your ability to think creatively.

Invigorating rosemary essential oil helps improve memory, wakefulness, and mood.

Notes and Tips:
You can make a larger batch of this blend to keep on hand by combining 50 drops grapefruit essential oil with 10 drops of rosemary essential oil in a 5 mL blue, green, or amber vial. Keep the blend by your bed and add it to your bedroom diffuser to help you wake up in the morning.

PART FOUR

Essential Oils for Cleaning

Kitchen and Bathroom Cleaning

ALL-PURPOSE CLEANER

Keeping your home clean is key in staying healthy, but most commercially available cleaning products are full of unhealthy ingredients. Natural cleaning solutions are generally safer for us and our families. When making your own cleaning products, you want ingredients that are simple and effective. This all-purpose cleaner is perfect for counter surfaces, floors, walls, and even toilets, sinks, and tubs. The best part about this cleaner, though, is that you can invite your children to clean with you. The essential oils contained in this recipe are safe for children ages two and older. You don't want them to drink it, of course, but spraying this while they help you clean won't irritate their little lungs like traditional cleaners will.

Ingredients:
½ cup white vinegar
1 ½ cup water
1 teaspoon Borax
10 drops lemon essential oil
5 drops melaleuca essential oil
5 drops lime essential oil
5 drops lemongrass essential oil
5 drops white fir essential oil

Preparation:
1. Use a metal funnel to combine all ingredients in 16-ounce blue or amber glass bottle.
2. Screw on a spray nozzle top.
3. Shake to mix ingredients thoroughly.

Administration:
1. Spray directly on the surface you wish to clean.
2. Use a cloth or natural sponge to scrub area and wipe clean.

Benefits:

Vinegar is often used alone as an effective natural disinfectant.

Borax reduces mold growth in both hard and porous surfaces. This is especially important when cleaning in the bathroom and kitchen.

Lemon, lemongrass, and melaleuca essential oils are all effective antimicrobials against multiple strains of staph, strep, and candida.

Lemongrass is particularly effective against listeria strains.

Citrus oils (including lemon and lime) contain limonene, which has a wide range of antimicrobial properties. These oils disinfect against food-related microorganisms, and have insecticidal properties as well. White fir essential oil also contains limonene.

Notes and Tips:

To increase the longevity of this cleaner, store it in a cool, dark place or even in the refrigerator.

If this spray gets in your or your child's eyes and is irritating, rinse with a carrier oil such as olive oil, sweet almond oil, or coconut oil. Do not rinse with water.

SANITIZING COUNTER SPRAY

Kitchen counters are one of the dirtiest places in our homes, even if they look clean. Food-borne pathogens are not visible to the naked eye and small splatters from uncooked meats and eggs, dairy products, and even fruits and vegetables can harbor harmful bacteria, viruses, and fungi. A safe cooking surface is paramount to serving healthy foods. The problem with most commercial cleaners for the kitchen is that they aren't safe to be used around food and definitely are not safe for ingestion. Warning labels tell you to make sure to clean any surfaces that will come in contact with food again after cleaning with those products. This kitchen counter spray is safe for cleaning your counters and for keeping your counter microbe free after you use it. Lemongrass and oregano essential oils are highly antimicrobial without damaging your lungs or skin. This spray leaves your kitchen smelling fresh and ready to use.

Ingredients:

½ cup white vinegar

1 ½ cup water

1 teaspoon Borax (optional)

25 drops lemongrass essential oil

15 drop oregano essential oil

Preparation:

1. Use a metal funnel to combine all ingredients in 16-ounce blue or amber glass bottle.
2. Screw on a spray nozzle top.
3. Shake to mix ingredients thoroughly.

Administration:

1. Spray directly onto your kitchen counter, refrigerator, or stove surfaces.
2. Use a cloth or natural sponge to scrub area and wipe clean.
3. If you do not include the borax, use the misting setting on the spray bottle nozzle to spray a fine mist over your countertops to protect the surfaces from contamination before you use them.

Benefits:

Both lemongrass and oregano essentials are highly effective against bacteria, viruses, and fungi including—but definitely not limited to—multiple strains of *listeria* (a common food-borne bacteria), *Escherichia coli, Salmonella enterica, Klebsiella pneumoniae, Acinetobacter baumannii, Pseudomonas aeruginosa, Enterococcus faecalis, Serratia marcescens, Staphylococcus aureus,* and *Candida albicans.* Many of the microbes inhibited by lemongrass and oregano essential oils have become drug-resistant, but not resistant to essential oils.

Lemongrass essential oil is one of the strongest antifungal essential oils.

Notes and Tips:

CAUTION: Oregano essential oil is not recommended for topical use in children under the age of six. It is safe to use this spray in areas where children will be, but it is not safe to let young children use this spray to clean. Instead, use the All-Purpose Cleaner (page 159).

If you do not have oregano essential oil, or want to add a festive touch to your counter spray, you can substitute cinnamon essential oil for the oregano.

Borax is not safe for ingestion in large doses, but is not harmful in the amount included in this spray. However, do not use borax in this recipe if food will come in contact with this spray.

CITRUS-FIR DISH SOAP

Properly washing dishes is an important part of preventing food-borne pathogens from contaminating our cooked food. This is especially true when washing cutting boards and other food prep materials. Essential oils are effective against many of the microbes that are carried in raw meats and unwashed fruits and vegetables. This dish soap cleans your dishes, kills microbes, and leaves your kitchen smelling pristine and uplifting.

Ingredients:
1 cup boiling water
¼ cup grated bar soap
¼ cup unscented liquid Castile soap
1 tablespoon washing soda (optional)
10 drops lemon essential oil
10 drops lemongrass essential oil
5 drops lime essential oil
5 drops white fir essential oil

Preparation:
1. Bring 1 cup water to a boil.
2. Turn off heat and add ¼ cup grated bar soap.
3. Stir until bar soap is melted into the water.
4. Add ¼ cup unscented liquid Castile soap.
5. Stir in 1 tablespoon washing soda (optional).
6. Use a funnel to pour the mixture into a 16-ounce blue or amber glass bottle.

7. Allow to cool.
8. Add 10 drops lemon, 10 drops lemongrass, 5 drops lime, and 5 drops white fir essential oils.
9. Cap with a pump top.
10. Shake well.

Administration:
1. Shake before using.
2. Wet dishes.
3. Pump out desired amount of Citrus-Fir Dish Soap onto a natural sponge.
4. Scrub dishes to remove food build up and grease.
5. Rinse dishes with hot water.
6. Air dry dishes in a dish rack or hand dry with a towel.

Benefits:
Lemongrass essential oil highly effective against bacteria, viruses, and fungi including multiple strains of *listeria* (a common food-borne bacteria), *Escherichia coli, Salmonella enterica, Klebsiella pneumoniae, Acinetobacter baumannii, Pseudomonas aeruginosa, Enterococcus faecalis, Serratia marcescens, Staphylococcus aureus,* and *Candida albicans.*

Lemon essential oil works both as a cleanser and a degreaser.

Lemon, lime, and white fir essential oils contain limonene, which has a wide range of antimicrobial properties, especially against food-borne pathogens.

Notes and Tips:
This dish soap is safe to use with children ages two and up who want to help out with washing the dishes. If you find that it irritates their skin, reduce the amount of lemon and lemongrass essential oils in the recipe to 5 drops each.

In colder months, use less washing soda or replace the washing soda with baking soda to prevent clogging of the dish soap pump.

Citrus-Fir Dish Soap is a part of the carpet cleaning protocol found on page 162.

GUNK- AND GREASE-REMOVING SPRAY

Oily gunk and grime can build up on kitchen surfaces quite quickly. Counter, stoves, ovens, stove hoods, refrigerators, floors, and even walls end up with splatter from cooking or mysterious sticky spots from who knows what. Soap and water, or even kitchen sprays, are hard pressed to remove all this residue. Surprisingly, the best solution is more oil! The slickness of olive oil, combined with the degreasing powers of lemon and eucalyptus essential oils, whisk away the gunk and grease that was so hard to get rid of before.

Ingredients:
⅓ cup olive oil
8 drops lemon essential oil
6 drops eucalyptus essential oil

Preparation:
1. Use a funnel to pour ⅓ cup olive oil into a 4-ounce blue or amber spray bottle.
2. Add 8 drops lemon and 6 drops eucalyptus essential oils.
3. Apply spray cap and shake well.

Administration:
1. Shake before using.
2. Spray the Gunk- and Grease-Removing Spray directly on any sticky, greasy, or gunky surfaces that need to be cleaned.
3. Allow to set for a few minutes and then use a cloth or natural sponge to remove spray and gunk from the soiled surface.

Benefits:
Limonene, found in lemon and other citrus essential oils, works as a solvent and degreaser.
The cineole in eucalyptus oil has industrial-strength grease solvent properties.

Notes and Tips:
This spray can also be used to remove grease from hands.

Store the Gunk- and Grease-Removing Spray in a cool, dry, and dark place to prevent the combination of oils from losing their efficacy or going rancid.

This spray is not intended for wood, carpet, or fabric surfaces.

BATHROOM SCRUB

Cleaning ourselves leads to having to clean our bathrooms regularly. Toilets, sinks, showers, and tubs get dirty from dust, water stains, beauty products, and even just daily use. Getting to these areas clean takes some elbow grease and a great cleaning product. Many commercial products are harsh on our lungs and leave us needing to shower to get them off our skin. This bathroom scrub is tough on dirt and stains, but gentle on your lungs and skin. It's even safe for children over the age of two to use when helping out with household cleaning.

Ingredients:

1 cup baking soda

1 cup witch hazel

8 drops lemon essential oil

6 drops geranium essential oil

6 drops melaleuca essential oil

4 drops orange essential oil

2 drops lemongrass essential oil

Preparation:

1. Pour 1 cup witch hazel into a 16-ounce wide-mouthed blue or amber bottle.
2. Add 8 drops lemon, 6 drops geranium, 6 drops melaleuca, 4 drops orange, and 2 drops lemongrass essential oils.
3. Swirl to combine.
4. Use a funnel to add 1 cup baking soda.
5. Cap with a powder-releasing cap.
6. Shake well to combine ingredients.

Administration:

1. Shake well before use.
2. Open the holes side of the powder-releasing cap.

3. Sprinkle the Bathroom Scrub over the area you desire to clean.
4. Use a scrub brush or sponge to clean the area.
5. Rinse with water.

Benefits:

Baking soda has long been used as a household cleaner. It gets rid of odors and acts as an abrasive to make scrubbing easier.

Lemon essential oil cuts oily buildup that can occur from using bath and beauty products.

Geranium, melaleuca, and lemongrass essential oils all deter fungal infections including athlete's foot. Making sure your shower/tub is free of this fungus is an important part of keeping your feet clean and healthy.

All the essential oils in this recipe are cleansing and antimicrobial.

Notes and Tips:

If you have hard water stains, spray the Sparkling Glass Cleaner (page 169), over the Bathroom Scrub. Let the scrub and spray combo set for 15 minutes and then use a natural scrub sponge to scrub away the hard water stains.

If you have a foot fungus infection, check out the Pedicure Prep Protocol (page 152) for keeping your feet fungus free.

LEMONGRASS-PEPPERMINT TOILET DROPS

When we use the restroom at home or as a guest, we don't want to leave unpleasant odors. Wouldn't it be great if the bathroom smelled better after we used it than it did before? Well, it's quite simple to achieve, actually. Simply use the Lemongrass-Peppermint Toilet drops before and after using the bathroom and leave the room smelling lovely.

Ingredients:

30 drops lemongrass essential oil
25 drops peppermint essential oil
10 drops geranium essential oil
5 drops basil essential oil

Preparation:

1. In a 5mL blue or amber vial, combine 30 drops lemongrass, 25 drops peppermint, 10 drops geranium, and 5 drops basil essential oils.
2. Place an orifice reducer in the mouth of the vial.
3. Apply a tight-fitting cap.
4. Shake well.

Administration:

1. Shake before use.
2. Before defecating in a toilet, add 3 drops of the Lemongrass-Peppermint Toilet Drops onto the surface of the toilet water.
3. Use the toilet.
4. Flush the toilet.
5. Add 3 more drops of the Lemongrass-Peppermint Toilet Drops to the surface of the toilet water and leave there until the toilet is used again.

Benefits:

Geranium essential oil is effective against airborne bacteria.

Toilet smells can come from contagious gut bacteria, viruses, and parasites. Lemongrass and basil essential oils protect against the spread of these microbes.

Lemongrass essential oil is particularly hearty at getting rid of stinky toilet smells.

The combination of peppermint and lemongrass essential oils leaves behind a pleasant aroma.

Notes and Tips:

Essential oils are hydrophobic so they stay on top of the toilet water's surface. This traps unpleasant odors underneath the essential oils.

If stored in a cool, dark, and dry location, the Peppermint-Lemongrass Toilet drops can be stored for up to a year.

AIR-FRESHENING DIFFUSER BLEND

There are a lot of reasons why your house—and especially your bathroom— might not smell so fresh. Funky smells can be caused by simply using the bathroom for its intended use, laundry that may be piling up, or even just having a teenager living in your house. Instead of just masking the odors with air sprays that aren't particularly good for your lungs, use the Air-Freshening Diffuser Blend to rid your bathroom—or other rooms!—of the sources of those odors.

Ingredients:
½ cup water
5 drops lemon essential oil
5 drops lime essential oil
2 drops melaleuca essential oil
2 drops lemongrass essential oil

Preparation:
1. Pour ½ cup water (or amount recommended for your particular diffuser) into your diffuser.
2. Add 5 drops each of lemon and lime essential oils.
3. Add 2 drops each of melaleuca and lemongrass essential oils.

Administration:
1. Place your diffuser on a flat surface near a plug in your bathroom.
2. Turn on the diffuser.

Benefits:
Lemon and lime essential oils cleanse the air.
Melaleuca and lemongrass essential oils get rid of mold and fungi that may
    be spreading through the air and causing unpleasant odors.
Lemongrass essential oil stamps out toilet-related odors.

Notes and Tips:
This blend can be used anywhere in the house that needs some freshening up.

   If you don't have a diffuser, you can add this blend (minus the water) to ½ a cup of baking soda in a 4-ounce mason jar. Just cover with a circle of fabric to create a simple jar air freshener.

SPARKLING GLASS CLEANER

Mirrors and glass surface can get just as gunky as countertops, but cleaning them can be a little bit harder. With glass, you have to be careful not to use regular oils that might leave streaking, which water can leave, too. Vinegar and essential oils are the perfect alternative solution due to quick evaporation, leaving your glass surfaces sparkling.

Ingredients:
1 ½ cups white vinegar
½ cup water
6 drops bergamot essential oil
6 drops lemon essential oil
6 drops orange essential oil

Preparation:
1. Use a funnel to pour 1 ½ cups white vinegar and ½ cup water into a 16-ounce blue of amber spray bottle.
2. Add 6 drops each of bergamot, lemon, and orange essential oils.
3. Cap with a spray nozzle.
4. Shake well to combine.

Administration:
1. Shake before use.
2. Spray the Sparkling Glass Cleaner onto any glass surface or mirror.
3. Wipe the area you want to clean with a lint-free towel.
4. Allow to air dry.

Benefits:
Citrus essential oils—including lemon, bergamot, and orange—are excellent degreasers and cleansers.
Vinegar cleans glass with a streak-free finish.

Notes and Tips:
Spray this over the Bathroom Scrub (page 165) to remove hard water stains.
Sparkling Glass Cleaning is a part of the Carpet Cleaning Protocol found on page 175.
This spray is safe for children over the age of two, who like to help with the chores—or are supposed to help with the chores!

Bedroom and Living Room Cleaning

DUSTING SPRAY

No matter how careful you are about spills, clutter, or tracking in a mess from outside, one household chore that will always need to be done is dusting. Dust comes from outside and inside your home and is a part of everyday living. However, wiping away dust and reducing its accumulation on household surfaces is made easier and more pleasant with this dusting spray.

Ingredients:
1 cup water
¼ cup vinegar
2 tablespoons olive oil
4 drops lemon essential oil
4 drops lemongrass essential oil
3 drops bergamot essential oil
3 drops lime essential oil

Preparation:
1. Use a funnel to pour 1 cup water into a 16-ounce blue or amber glass spray bottle.
2. Once again use the funnel to add ¼ cup vinegar.
3. Add 2 tablespoons olive oil.
4. Add 4 drops each lemon and lemongrass essential oils.
5. Add 3 drops each bergamot and lime essential oils.
6. Top with a spray nozzle.
7. Shake well.

Administration:
1. Shake well before using.

2. Spray onto a microfiber cloth.
3. Wipe down areas that accumulate dust to remove the dust and prevent future buildup.

Benefits:
Lemon essential oil and vinegar both cut through grease.

Olive oil protects wood surfaces and prevents dust from settling on surfaces.

Lemongrass essential oil is highly antimicrobial and cleans the surfaces you are dusting.

Citrus oils—such as lemon, bergamot, and lime—are cleansing and also mood enhancing. This makes the chore of dusting a little more pleasant.

Notes and Tips:
Almond oil or avocado oil can be substituted for the olive oil.

Grapefruit or orange essential oils may be substituted for the bergamot or lime essential oils.

MATTRESS-CLEANING POWDER

When we clean our home, we often leave our mattresses out of the equation. We may flip them every six months and change the sheets regularly, but unless they get a particular stain or infestation, we generally leave our mattresses alone. This means our mattresses can become quite dirty without us even realizing it. We can't throw our mattresses in the washer and dryer and a steam cleaned mattress takes forever to dry. Instead, use the Mattress-Cleaning Powder for a dry freshening and cleaning of your mattress.

Ingredients:
2 cups baking soda, divided
9 drops lavender essential oil, divided
6 drops ylang-ylang essential oil, divided
6 drops clove essential oil, divided
3 drops cedarwood essential oil, divided

Preparation:

1. Pour ½ cup baking soda into a 16-ounce, wide-mouthed bottle.
2. Add 3 drops lavender, 2 drops ylang-ylang, 2 drops clove, and 1 drop cedarwood essential oils.
3. Add 1 cup baking soda.
4. Add 3 drops lavender, 2 drops ylang-ylang, 2 drops clove, and 1 drop cedarwood essential oils.
5. Add the last ½ cup baking soda.
6. Add the final 3 drops lavender, 2 drops ylang-ylang, 2 drops clove, and 1 drop cedarwood essential oils.
7. Top with a powder dispensing lid.

Administration:

1. Sprinkle the Mattress-Cleaning Powder over your bare mattress.
2. Let stand for an hour or two.
3. Vacuum up the Mattress-Cleaning Powder from the bed.

Benefits:

Baking soda cleans the mattress, absorbs moisture, and stamps out odors.
Lavender essential oil contains linalool, which helps you sleep better at night.
Ylang-ylang essential oil also has a calming effect and promotes sleep.
Clove essential oil cleans your mattress by eradicating any bacteria, viruses, or fungi that may be lingering in your mattress.
Lavender, cedarwood, and clove essential oils can repel insects.
Ylang-ylang essential oil protects against dust mites.

Notes and Tips:

Use the Mattress-Cleaning Powder if you or your partner are sick to reduce the risk of the other person getting sick, too.

Use the Mattress-Cleaning Powder as a part of the Carpet Cleaning Protocol found on page 175.

CITRUS CLEAN LAUNDRY DETERGENT

Laundry detergent can get expensive, and it's an item we have to buy on a regular basis. Making your own laundry detergent out of simple ingredients and essential oils is not only less expensive, but better for you and the environment. You can still get the amazing clean you're looking for with the Citrus Clean Laundry Detergent, plus you have the added benefit of your detergent being antifungal to keep mildew away.

Ingredients:
1 cup super washing soda
1 cup borax
5 ounces pure Castile soap, grated
20 drops bergamot essential oil
20 drops lemon essential oil
20 drops orange essential oil
10 drops basil essential oil
10 drops melaleuca essential oil

Preparation:
1. Finely grate one bar (5 ounces) of pure Castile soap into a large glass bowl.
2. Add 1 cup each of super washing soda and borax.
3. Stir well to mix.
4. Add 20 drops each of bergamot, lemon, and orange essential oils.
5. Stir well to mix.
6. Add 10 drops each basil and melaleuca essential oils.
7. Stir well to mix.
8. Store in a 20-ounce, wide-mouth glass jar.

Administration:
1. Fill your washing machine with water.
2. Add ¼ cup Citrus Clean Laundry Detergent.
3. Close the lid for 10–15 seconds to allow the detergent to mix with the water.
4. Add your laundry.
5. Close lid and let laundry cycle complete.

Benefits:
Basil essential oil contains methyl chavicol, linalool, eugenol, and eucalyptol, which all significantly reduce the growth of mildew.

In addition to being antifungal, linalool is a mood-lifting component of several essential oils. Orange and bergamot essential oils also contain linalool.

Like linalool, limonene is uplifting and antifungal. Limonene is found in all the citrus essential oils such as orange, lemon, and bergamot. Limonene has the added benefit of being chemopreventive—protecting against cancer—specifically against breast cancer.

Terpinen-4-ol, found in melaleuca essential oil, protects against many of the fungal infections that affect humans.

Notes and Tips:

If you are washing clothes for children under the age of two, omit the basil essential oil.

For children over the age of two, the bergamot, lemon, and orange essential oils can be substituted with grapefruit or lime essential oils, which also contain limonene.

If your laundry accidentally gets left in the washing machine, add 1 drop of lemongrass essential oil to the laundry detergent when you run the laundry through the wash again.

LAVENDER-ORANGE DRYER SHEETS

One of the wonderful parts of taking your clean clothes out of the dryer is feeling their warmth and smelling their fresh clean, scent. Taking a deep breath to inhale that beautiful smell is even better when you've been using these Lavender-Orange Dryer Sheets. Your clothes will relax you, and wearing them will improve your day.

Ingredients:
reusable wipes (or dry washcloth)
1 drop lavender essential oil
1 drop orange essential oil

Preparation:
1. Place 1 drop each of lavender and orange essential oil on a reusable wipe (or dry washcloth).

Administration:
1. Place dryer sheet in the dryer with your laundry.
2. Set dryer to desired settings.
3. Turn on dryer.
4. Remove dryer sheet with your laundry and save for future use.

Benefits:
Lavender and orange essential oils help to continue to clean your clothes while they are in the dryer.

Lavender essential oil relaxes your mind and body.

Orange essential oil improves your mood.

Notes and Tips:
Reuse the reusable wipe to make new dryer sheets for your next load.

Drying your clothes, if possible, on lower settings keeps your clothes from wearing down and maintains the scent of the essential oils better.

CARPET CLEANING PROTOCOL

Keeping your carpet clean can be a difficult battle. Spilled drinks, pet stains, children being children, foot traffic, and daily life all contribute to carpet stains. Hauling out a carpet cleaner or hiring a carpet cleaning company is cumbersome and gets expensive. Instead, take care of your carpet yourself with this carpet cleaning protocol. Your carpet will practically sparkle and your house will smell amazing.

Ingredients:
Citrus-Fir Dish Soap (pg 162)
Mattress-Cleaning Powder (pg 171)
Sparkling Glass Cleaner (pg 169)

Administration:
1. Use the Citrus-Fir Dish Soap to scrub any visible stains on the carpet.
2. Sprinkle the Mattress-Cleaning Powder over the carpet.
3. Spray the Sparkling Glass Cleaner over the Mattress-Cleaning Powder.

4. Allow the carpet cleaning mixture to set and dry.
5. Vacuum it up.

Benefits:

The baking soda in the Mattress-Cleaning Powder and the vinegar in the Sparking Class Cleaner work together to lift stains.

The citrus oils, along with the lemongrass and clove essential oils, in this protocol clean your carpet. They affect bacteria, viruses, and fungi.

The lemongrass essential oil in the Citrus-Fir Dish Soap is particularly effective against molds and mildew.

The lavender, clove, and cedarwood in the Mattress-Cleaning Powder help to repel insects that may want to come into your home.

Notes and Tips:

If you do not have any visible stains on your carpet, you can skip using the Citrus-Fir Dish Soap for this protocol.

Be sure to start vacuuming with a clean filter in your vacuum.

References

Acharya, Asha, Ila Das, Sushmita Singh, and Tapas Saha. "Chemopreventive properties of indole-3-carbinol, diindolylmethane and other constituents of cardamom against carcinogenesis." *Recent patents on food, nutrition & agriculture* 2, no. 2 (2010): 166–177.

Adsersen, Anne, Bente Gauguin, Lene Gudiksen, and Anna K. Jäger. "Screening of plants used in Danish folk medicine to treat memory dysfunction for acetylcholinesterase inhibitory activity." *Journal of Ethnopharmacology* 104, no. 3 (2006): 418–422.

Agarwal, Ruchika. "Eucalyptus oil in dentistry: A mini Review." *Int. J. Drug Dev. & Res* 5, no. 4 (2013): 0975–9344.

Akkol, Esra Küpeli, Ayşegül Güvenç, and Erdem Yesilada. "A comparative study on the antinociceptive and anti-inflammatory activities of five Juniperus taxa." *Journal of ethnopharmacology* 125, no. 2 (2009): 330–336.

Al-Harrasi, Ahmed, and Salim Al-Saidi. "Phytochemical analysis of the essential oil from botanically certified oleogum resin of Boswellia sacra (Omani Luban)."*Molecules* 13, no. 9 (2008): 2181–2189.

Al-Waili, N. S. (2003). Topical application of natural honey, beeswax, and olive oil mixture for atopic dermatitis or psoriasis: partially controlled, single-blinded study. *Complementary therapies in medicine*, *11*(4), 226–234.

Alankar, Shrivastava. "A review on peppermint oil." *Asian Journal of Pharmaceutical and Clinical Research* 2, no. 2 (2009): 27–33.

Anilkumar, M. "10. Ethnomedicinal plants as anti-inflammatory and analgesic agents." *Ethnomedicine: A Source of Complementary Therapeutics*, (2010): 267–293

Ankri, Serge, and David Mirelman. "Antimicrobial properties of allicin from garlic." *Microbes and infection* 1.2 (1999): 125–129.

Anstey, A., M. Quigley, and J. D. Wilkinson. "Topical evening primrose oil as treatment for atopic eczema." *Journal of Dermatological Treatment* 1, no. 4 (1990): 199–201.

Anthony, Jean-Paul, Lorna Fyfe, and Huw Smith. "Plant active components–a resource for antiparasitic agents?." *Trends in parasitology* 21, no. 10 (2005): 462–468.

Arias, Beatriz Alvarez, and Luis Ramón-Laca. "Pharmacological properties of citrus and their ancient and medieval uses in the Mediterranean region." *Journal of Ethnopharmacology* 97, no. 1 (2005): 89–95.

Arnett, Frank C., Steven M. Edworthy, Daniel A. Bloch, Dennis J. Mcshane, James F. Fries, Norman S. Cooper, Louis A. Healey et al. "The American Rheumatism Association 1987 revised criteria for the classification of rheumatoid arthritis." *Arthritis & Rheumatism* 31, no. 3 (1988): 315–324.

Asha'ari, Zamzil Amin, Mohd Zaki Ahmad, Wan Din, Wan Shah Jihan, Che Hussin, Che Maraina, and Wan Ishlah Leman. "Ingestion of honey improves the symptoms of allergic rhinitis: Evidence from a randomized placebo-controlled trial in the East Coast of Peninsular Malaysia." *Annals of Saudi medicine* 33, no. 5 (2013): 469–475.

Athar, Mohammad, and Syed Mahmood Nasir. "Taxonomic perspective of plant species yielding vegetable oils used in cosmetics and skin care products." *African Journal of Biotechnology* 4, no. 1 (2005).

Ayedoun, Abel Marc, Bouraïman Salami Adeoti, Jacques Setondji, Chantal Menut, Gérard Lamaty, and Jean-Marie Bessiére. "Aromatic plants from Tropical West Africa. IV. Chemical composition of leaf oil of Pimenta racemosa (Miller) JW Moore var. racemosa from Benin." *Journal of Essential Oil Research* 8, no. 2 (1996): 207–209.

Badmaev, Vladimir, Muhammed Majeed, and Lakshmi Prakash. "Piperine derived from black pepper increases the plasma levels of coenzyme Q10 following oral supplementation." *The journal of nutritional biochemistry* 11, no. 2 (2000): 109–113.

Bağci, Eyüp, and Metin Diğrak. "Antimicrobial activity of essential oils of some Abies (Fir) species from Turkey." *Flavour and fragrance journal* 11.4 (1996): 251–256.

Bagetta, Giacinto, Luigi Antonio Morrone, Laura Rombolà, Diana Amantea, Rossella Russo, Laura Berliocchi, Shinobu Sakurada, Tsukasa Sakurada, Domenicantonio Rotiroti, and Maria Tiziana Corasaniti. "Neuropharmacology of the essential oil of bergamot." *Fitoterapia* 81, no. 6 (2010): 453–461.

Balakrishnan, K. P., and Nithya Narayanaswamy. "Botanicals as sunscreens: their role in the prevention of photoaging and skin cancer." *Int. J. Cosmetic Sci* 1, no. 1 (2011): 1–12.

Barnard, D. R. "GLOBAL COLLABORATION FOR DEVELOPMENT OF PESTICIDES FOR PUBLIC HEALTH." World Health Organization (2000).

Basch, Ethan, Catherine Ulbricht, Paul Hammerness, Anja Bevins, and David Sollars. "Thyme (Thymus vulgaris L.), thymol." *Journal of herbal pharmacotherapy* 4, no. 1 (2004): 49–67.

Bell, Kristen Leigh. *Holistic Aromatherapy for Animals: A Comprehensive Guide to Using Essential Oils and Hydrosols with Dogs, Cats, Horses and Other Animals*. Findhorn Press, 2002.

Bender, Tamás, Zeki Karagülle, Géza P. Bálint, Christoph Gutenbrunner, Péter V. Bálint, and Shaul Sukenik. "Hydrotherapy, balneotherapy, and spa treatment in pain management." *Rheumatology international* 25, no. 3 (2005): 220–224.

Bennett, Richard N., and Roger M. Wallsgrove. "Tansley Review No. 72. Secondary metabolites in plant defence mechanisms." *New Phytologist* (1994): 617–633.

Benor, Daniel J., and ABIHM IJHC. "Complementary therapies for Attention Deficit Hyperactivity Disorder (ADHD)." *Int J Heal Caring* 6 (2006): 1–15.

Bommareddy, Ajay, Brittny Rule, Adam L. VanWert, Sreevidya Santha, and Chandradhar Dwivedi. "α-Santalol, a derivative of sandalwood oil, induces apoptosis in human prostate cancer cells by causing caspase-3 activation."*Phytomedicine* 19, no. 8 (2012): 804–811.

Bordoni, A., P. L. Biagi, M. Masi, G. Ricci, C. Fanelli, A. Patrizi, and E. Ceccolini. "Evening primrose oil (Efamol) in the treatment of children with atopic eczema." *Drugs under experimental and clinical research* 14, no. 4 (1987): 291–297.

Brown, Sylvia T., Carol Douglas, and LeeAnn Plaster Flood. "Women's evaluation of intrapartum nonpharmacological pain relief methods used during labor." *The journal of perinatal education* 10, no. 3 (2001): 1.

Buchbauer, G. "Evaluation of the effects of East Indian sandalwood oil and α-santalol on humans after transdermal absorption." *Planta Med* 70 (2004): 3–7.

Buchbauer, Gerhard. "East Indian sandalwood and α-santalol odor increase physiological and self-rated arousal in humans." *Planta Med* 72 (2006): 792–800.

Burks-Wicks, Carla, Misha Cohen, Josef Fallbacher, Robert N Taylor, and Fritz Wieser. "A Western primer of Chinese herbal therapy in endometriosis and infertility." (2005): 447–463.

Burns, E., Blamey, C., Ersser, S. J., Lloyd, A. J., & Barnetson, L. (2000). The use of aromatherapy in intrapartum midwifery practice an observational study. *Complementary therapies in nursing & midwifery*, 6(1), 33.

Burrello, Nunziatina, Aldo E. Calogero, Anna Perdichizzi, Mario Salmeri, Rosario D'Agata, and Enzo Vicari. "Inhibition of oocyte fertilization by assisted reproductive techniques and increased sperm DNA fragmentation in the presence of Candida albicans: a case report." *Reproductive biomedicine online* 8, no. 5 (2004): 569–573.

Burt, Sara A., and Robert D. Reinders. "Antibacterial activity of selected plant essential oils against Escherichia coli O157: H7." *Letters in applied microbiology* 36, no. 3 (2003): 162–167.

Bush, L. J., J. D. Schuh, N. B. Tennille, and G. R. Waller. "Effect of dietary fat and minerals on the incidence of diarrhea and rate of passage of diets in the digestive tract of dairy calves." *Journal of Dairy Science* 46, no. 7 (1963): 703–709.

Carbajal, D., Molina, V., Valdés, S., Arruzazabala, M. D. L., Más, R., & Magraner, J. (1998). Anti-inflammatory activity of D-002: an active product isolated from beeswax. *Prostaglandins, Leukotrienes and Essential fatty acids,59*(4), 235–238.

Carlson, Luiz Henrique Castelan, Ariovaldo Bolzan, and Ricardo Antônio Francisco Machado. "Separation of d-limonene from supercritical CO 2 by means of membranes." The Journal of supercritical fluids 34, no. 2 (2005): 143–147.

Carrasco, Fábio Ricardo, Gustavo Schmidt, Adriano Lopez Romero, Juliano Luiz Sartoretto, Silvana Martins Caparroz-Assef, Ciomar Aparecida Bersani-Amado, and Roberto Kenji Nakamura Cuman. "Immunomodulatory activity of Zingiber officinale Roscoe, Salvia officinalis L. and Syzygium aromaticum L. essential oils: evidence for humor- and cell-mediated responses." *Journal of Pharmacy and Pharmacology* 61, no. 7 (2009): 961–967.

Cassella, S., John P. Cassella, and I. Smith. "Synergistic antifungal activity of tea tree (Melaleuca alternifolia) and lavender (Lavandula angustifolia) essential oils against dermatophyte infection." *International Journal of Aromatherapy* 12, no. 1 (2002): 2–15.

Cavanagh, H. M. A., and J. M. Wilkinson. "Biological activities of lavender essential oil." *Phytotherapy Research* 16, no. 4 (2002): 301–308.

Ceccarelli, Ilaria, William R. Lariviere, Paolo Fiorenzani, Paola Sacerdote, and Anna Maria Aloisi. "Effects of long-term exposure of lemon essential oil odor on behavioral, hormonal and neuronal parameters in male and female rats." *Brain research* 1001, no. 1 (2004): 78–86.

Chaieb, Kamel, Hafedh Hajlaoui, Tarek Zmantar, Amel Ben Kahla Nakbi, Mahmoud Rouabhia, Kacem Mahdouani, and Amina Bakhrouf. "The chemical composition and biological activity of clove essential oil, Eugenia caryophyllata (Syzigium aromaticum L. Myrtaceae): a short review." *Phytotherapy research* 21, no. 6 (2007): 501–506.

Chang, Kang-Ming, and Chuh-Wei Shen. "Aromatherapy benefits autonomic nervous system regulation for elementary school faculty in Taiwan." *Evidence-Based Complementary and Alternative Medicine* 2011 (2011).

Chanthaphon, Sumonrat, Suphitchaya Chanthachum, and Tipparat Hongpattarakere. "Antimicrobial activities of essential oils and crude extracts from tropical Citrus spp. against food-related microorganisms." *Sonklanakarin Journal of Science and Technology* 30.1 (2008): 125.

Chao, Sue C., D. Gary Young, and Craig J. Oberg. "Screening for inhibitory activity of essential oils on selected bacteria, fungi and viruses." *Journal of Essential Oil Research* 12, no. 5 (2000): 639–649.

Chen, Jaw-Chyun, Li-Jiau Huang, Shih-Lu Wu, Sheng-Chu Kuo, Tin-Yun Ho, and Chien-Yun Hsiang. "Ginger and its bioactive component inhibit enterotoxigenic Escherichia coli heat-labile enterotoxin-induced diarrhea in mice." *Journal of agricultural and food chemistry* 55, no. 21 (2007): 8390–8397.

Choi, Hyang-Sook, Hee Sun Song, Hiroyuki Ukeda, and Masayoshi Sawamura. "Radical-scavenging activities of citrus essential oils and their components: detection using 1, 1-diphenyl-2-picrylhydrazyl." *Journal of agricultural and food chemistry* 48, no. 9 (2000): 4156–4161.

Chrubasik, S., M. H. Pittler, and B. D. Roufogalis. "Zingiberis rhizoma: a comprehensive review on the ginger effect and efficacy profiles." *Phytomedicine* 12, no. 9 (2005): 684–701.

Chu, Catherine J., and Kathi J. Kemper. "Lavender (Lavandula spp.)." *Longwood Herbal Task Force. 32p* (2001).

Cioanca, Oana, Lucian Hritcu, Marius Mihasan, Adriana Trifan, and Monica Hancianu. "Inhalation of coriander volatile oil increased anxiolytic-antidepressant-like behaviors and decreased oxidative status in beta-amyloid (1–42) rat model of Alzheimer's disease." *Physiology & behavior* 131 (2014): 68–74.

Clark, E. W., & Steel, I. (1993). Investigations into biomechanisms of moisturizing function of lanolin. *JOURNAL-SOCIETY OF COSMETIC CHEMISTS*, *44*, 181.

Clark, Kerry L., and Lance A. Durden. "Parasitic arthropods of small mammals in Mississippi." *Journal of Mammalogy* 83, no. 4 (2002): 1039–1048

Cox, S. D., C. M. Mann, J. L. Markham, H. C. Bell, J. E. Gustafson, J. R. Warmington, and S. G. Wyllie. "The mode of antimicrobial action of the essential oil of Melaleuca alternifolia (tea tree oil)." *Journal of applied microbiology* 88, no. 1 (2000): 170–175.

Damian, Peter. *Aromatherapy: Scent and Psyche: Using Essential Oils for Physical and Emotional Well-Being*. Inner Traditions/Bear & Co, 1995.

Dave, Vivek, and Sachdev Yadav. "Aromatherapy for stress relief." *International Journal of Research and Development in Pharmacy and Life Sciences* 2, No.3 (2013) 398–403.

Davis, John B., Julie Gray, Martin J. Gunthorpe, Jonathan P. Hatcher, Phil T. Davey, Philip Overend, Mark H. Harries et al. "Vanilloid receptor-1 is essential for inflammatory thermal hyperalgesia." *Nature* 405, no. 6783 (2000): 183–187.

de Almeida, Igor, Daniela Sales Alviano, Danielle Pereira Vieira, Péricles Barreto Alves, Arie Fitzgerald Blank, Angela Hampshire CS Lopes, Celuta Sales Alviano, and S. Rosa Maria do Socorro. "Antigiardial activity of Ocimum basilicum essential oil." *Parasitology research* 101, no. 2 (2007): 443–452.

Della Ragione, Fulvio, Valeria Cucciolla, Adriana Borriello, Valentina Della Pietra, Gabriele Pontoni, Luigi Racioppi, Caterina Manna, Patrizia Galletti, and Vincenzo Zappia. "Hydroxytyrosol, a natural molecule occurring in olive oil, induces cytochrome c-dependent apoptosis." *Biochemical and biophysical research communications* 278, no. 3 (2000): 733–739.

Dhang, Partho, and K. Purusotaman Sanjayan. "15 Plants with Pest Control Properties Against Urban Pests." *Urban Insect Pests: Sustainable Management Strategies* (2014): 216.

Dharmananda, Subhuti. *Chinese Herbal Therapy for Endometriosis.* ITM, 2002.

Dharmananda, Subhuti. *Treatment of interstitial cystitis with Chinese medicine.* ITM, 2003.

Diego, Miguel A., Nancy Aaron Jones, Tiffany Field, Maria Hernandez-Reif, Saul Schanberg, Cynthia Kuhn, Mary Galamaga, Virginia McAdam, and Robert Galamaga. "Aromatherapy positively affects mood, EEG patterns of alertness and math computations." *International Journal of Neuroscience* 96, no. 3–4 (1998): 217–224.

Dobetsberger, Clara, and Gerhard Buchbauer. "Actions of essential oils on the central nervous system: An updated review." *Flavour and Fragrance Journal* 26, no. 5 (2011): 300–316.

Dorman, H. J. D., and S. G. Deans. "Antimicrobial agents from plants: antibacterial activity of plant volatile oils." *Journal of applied microbiology* 88, no. 2 (2000): 308–316.

Dougans, Inge and Suzanne Ellis. *The Art of Reflexology: A Step-by-Step Guide.* Element, 1992.

Dwivedi, C., and A. Abu-Ghazaleh. "Chemopreventive effects of sandalwood oil on skin papillomas in mice." *European journal of cancer prevention* 6, no. 4 (1997): 399–401.

Dwivedi, C., and Y. Zhang. "Sandalwood oil prevents skin tumour development in CD1 mice." *European journal of cancer prevention* 8, no. 5 (1999): 449–456.

Edris, Amr E. "Pharmaceutical and therapeutic potentials of essential oils and their individual volatile constituents: a review." *Phytotherapy Research* 21, no. 4 (2007): 308–323.

Edwards-Jones, Valerie, Rachael Buck, Susan G. Shawcross, Maureen M. Dawson, and Ken Dunn. "The effect of essential oils on methicillin-resistant Staphylococcus aureus using a dressing model." *Burns* 30, no. 8 (2004): 772–777.

El Ashry, E. S. H., Rashed, N., Salama, O. M., & Saleh, A. (2003). Components, therapeutic value and uses of myrrh. *Die Pharmazie-An International Journal of Pharmaceutical Sciences*, 58(3), 163–168.

El-Ashmawy, Ibrahim M., Amal Saleh, and Osama M. Salama. "Effects of marjoram volatile oil and grape-seed extract on ethanol toxicity in male rats."*Basic & clinical pharmacology & toxicology* 101, no. 5 (2007): 320–327.

Elisabetsky, Elaine, Jeanine Marschner, and Diogo Onofre Souza. "Effects of linalool on glutamatergic system in the rat cerebral cortex." *Neurochemical research* 20, no. 4 (1995): 461–465.

Fakari, Fahimeh Rashidi, Mahbubeh Tabatabaeichehr, Hossian Kamali, Farzaneh Rashidi Fakari, and Maryam Naseri. "Effect of Inhalation of Aroma of Geranium Essence on Anxiety and Physiological Parameters during First Stage of Labor in Nulliparous Women: a Randomized Clinical Trial." *Journal of Caring Sciences* 4, no. 2 (2015): 135–141.

Farnan, T. B., J. McCallum, A. Awa, A. D. Khan, and S. J. Hall. "Tea tree oil: in vitro efficacy in otitis externa." *Journal of Laryngology & Otology* 119, no. 03 (2005): 198–201.

Fayed, Sayed A. "Antioxidant and anticancer activities of Citrus reticulate (Petitgrain Mandarin) and Pelargonium graveolens (Geranium) essential oils."*Research Journal of Agriculture and Biological Sciences* 5, no. 5 (2009): 740–747.

Field, Tiffany, M. Hemandez-Reif, Steven Taylor, O. Quintino, and I. Burman. "Labor pain is reduced by massage therapy." *Journal of Psychosomatic Obstetrics & Gynecology* 18, no. 4 (1997): 286–291.

Field, Tiffany, Miguel Diego, Maria Hernandez-Reif, and Jean Shea. "Hand arthritis pain is reduced by massage therapy." *Journal of Bodywork and Movement Therapies* 11, no. 1 (2007): 21–24.

Fingerova, H., I. Oborna, P. Petrova, M. Budikova, and J. Jezdínský. "[Does grapefruit juice increase the bioavailability of orally administered sex steroids?]."*Ceska gynekologie/Ceska lekarska spolecnost J. Ev. Purkyne* 68, no. 2 (2003): 117–121.

Fitó, Montserrat, Rafael de la Torre, Magi Farré-Albaladejo, Olha Khymenetz, Jaime Marrugat, and Maria-Isabel Covas. "Bioavailability and antioxidant effects of olive oil phenolic compounds in humans: a review." *Annali dell'Istituto superiore di sanitÃ* 43, no. 4 (2006): 375–381.

Fradelos, E., and A. Komini. "The use of essential oils as a complementary treatment for anxiety." *American Journal of Nursing* 4.1 (2015): 1–5.

Francisco, Vera, Artur Figueirinha, Gustavo Costa, Joana Liberal, Maria Celeste Lopes, Carmen García-Rodríguez, Carlos FGC Geraldes, Maria T. Cruz, and Maria T. Batista. "Chemical characterization and anti-inflammatory activity of luteolin glycosides isolated from lemongrass." *Journal of Functional Foods* 10 (2014): 436–443.

Friedman, Mendel, Philip R. Henika, and Robert E. Mandrell. "Bactericidal activities of plant essential oils and some of their isolated constituents against Campylobacter jejuni, Escherichia coli, Listeria monocytogenes, and Salmonella enterica." *Journal of Food Protection*® 65, no. 10 (2002): 1545–1560.

Friedman, Mendel, Philip R. Henika, Carol E. Levin, and Robert E. Mandrell. "Antibacterial activities of plant essential oils and their components against Escherichia coli O157: H7 and Salmonella enterica in apple juice." *Journal of agricultural and food chemistry* 52, no. 19 (2004): 6042–6048.

Fu, YuJie, YuanGang Zu, LiYan Chen, XiaoGuang Shi, Zhe Wang, Su Sun, and Thomas Efferth. "Antimicrobial activity of clove and rosemary essential oils alone and in combination." *Phytotherapy Research* 21, no. 10 (2007): 989–994.

Fukumoto, Syuichi, Aya Morishita, Kohei Furutachi, Takehiko Terashima, Tsutomu Nakayama, and Hidehiko Yokogoshi. "Effect of flavour components in lemon essential oil on physical or psychological stress." *Stress and Health* 24, no. 1 (2008): 3–12.

Gardner, D. R., K. E. Panter, L. F. James, and B. L. Stegelmeier. "Abortifacient effects of lodgepole pine (Pinus contorta) and common juniper (Juniperus communis) on cattle." *Veterinary and human toxicology* 40, no. 5 (1998): 260–263.

Gattefosse, Rene Maurice. *Gattefosse's aromatherapy*. Random House, 2012.

Gedney, Jeffrey J., Toni L. Glover, and Roger B. Fillingim. "Sensory and affective pain discrimination after inhalation of essential oils." *Psychosomatic Medicine* 66, no. 4 (2004): 599–606.

Geiger, James L. "The essential oil of ginger, Zingiber officinale, and anaesthesia." *International Journal of Aromatherapy* 15, no. 1 (2005): 7–14.

Genovese, Allison G., Mary Kay McLean, and Safdar A. Khan. "Adverse reactions from essential oil-containing natural flea products exempted from

Environmental Protection Agency regulations in dogs and cats." *Journal of Veterinary Emergency and Critical Care* 22, no. 4 (2012): 470–475.

Göbel, H., G. Schmidt, and D. Soyka. "Effect of peppermint and eucalyptus oil preparations on neurophysiological and experimental algesimetric headache parameters." *Cephalalgia* 14, no. 3 (1994): 228–234.

Goes, Tiago Costa, Fabrício Dias Antunes, Péricles Barreto Alves, and Flavia Teixeira-Silva. "Effect of sweet orange aroma on experimental anxiety in humans." *The Journal of Alternative and Complementary Medicine* 18, no. 8 (2012): 798–804.

Guillaume, Dom, and Zoubida Charrouf. "Argan oil." *Alternative Medicine Review* 16, no. 3 (2011): 275–279.

Gwaltney Jr, J. M., A. Sydnor Jr, and M. A. Sande. "Etiology and antimicrobial treatment of acute sinusitis." *The Annals of otology, rhinology & laryngology. Supplement* 90, no. 3 Pt 3 (1980): 68–71.

Hammer, Katherine A., C. F. Carson, and T. V. Riley. "Antimicrobial activity of essential oils and other plant extracts." *Journal of applied microbiology* 86, no. 6 (1999): 985–990.

Hanuš, L. O., T. Řezanka, V. M. Dembitsky, and A. Moussaieff. "Myrrh-commiphora chemistry." *Biomedical papers*, *149*, no. 1(2005), 3–28.

Hay, Isabelle C., Margaret Jamieson, and Anthony D. Ormerod. "Randomized trial of aromatherapy: successful treatment for alopecia areata." *Archives of dermatology* 134, no. 11 (1998): 1349–1352.

Heinrich, U., H. Tronnier, W. Stahl, M. Bejot, and J. M. Maurette. "Antioxidant supplements improve parameters related to skin structure in humans." *Skin pharmacology and physiology* 19, no. 4 (2006): 224–231.

Hendel, Barbara, and Peter Ferreira. "Water and Salt, the Essence of Life." *Natural Resources* (2003): 251.

Herman, A., and A. P. Herman. "Caffeine's mechanisms of action and its cosmetic use." *Skin pharmacology and physiology* 26, no. 1 (2012): 8–14.

Hink, W. F., T. A. Liberati, and M. G. Collart. "Toxicity of linalool to life stages of the cat flea, Ctenocephalides felis (Siphonaptera: Pulicidae), and its efficacy in carpet and on animals." *Journal of medical entomology* 25, no. 1 (1988): 1–4.

Hire, Kushal K., and D. A. Dhale. "ANTIMICROBIAL EFFECT AND INSILICO ADMET PREDICTION OF SANTALUM ALBUM L." *International Journal of Pharma and Bio Sciences* 3.4 (2012): 727–734.

Holmes, Peter. "Uplifting oils: The treatment of depression in clinical aromatherapy." *International Journal of Aromatherapy* 9, no. 3 (1999): 102–104.

Hongratanaworakit, Tapanee, and Gerhard Buchbauer. "Relaxing effect of ylang-ylang oil on humans after transdermal absorption." *Phytotherapy Research* 20, no. 9 (2006): 758–763.

Hosseini, Mahmoud, Mina Kamkar Asl, and Hassan Rakhshandeh. "Analgesic effect of clove essential oil in mice." *Avicenna Journal of Phytomedicine* 1, no. 1 (2011): 1–6.

Hur, Myung-Haeng, Myeong Soo Lee, Ka-Yeon Seong, and Mi-Kyoung Lee. "Aromatherapy massage on the abdomen for alleviating menstrual pain in high school girls: a preliminary controlled clinical study." *Evidence-Based Complementary and Alternative Medicine* 2012 (2011).

Hwang, Jin Hee. "[The effects of the inhalation method using essential oils on blood pressure and stress responses of clients with essential hypertension]." *Taehan Kanho Hakhoe Chi* 36, no. 7 (2006): 1123–1134.

Ibrahim, Mohamed A., Pirjo Kainulainen, and Abbas Aflatuni. "Insecticidal, repellent, antimicrobial activity and phytotoxicity of essential oils: with special reference to limonene and its suitability for control of insect pests." *Agricultural and Food Science* 10.3 (2008): 243–259.

Infante, Rodrigo, Pia Rubio, Loreto Contador, and Violeta Moreno. "Effect of drying process on lemon verbena (Lippia citrodora Kunth) aroma and infusion sensory quality." *International journal of food science & technology* 45, no. 1 (2010): 75–80.

Inoue, Toshio, Yukio Sugimoto, Hideki Masuda, and Chiaki Kamei. "Effects of peppermint (Mentha piperita L.) extracts on experimental allergic rhinitis in rats." *Biological and Pharmaceutical Bulletin* 24, no. 1 (2001): 92–95.

Inouye, Shigeharu, Katsuhisa Uchida, Yayoi Nishiyama, Yayoi Hasumi, Hideyo Yamaguchi, and Shigeru Abe. "Combined effect of heat, essential oils and salt on the fungicidal activity against Trichophyton mentagrophytes in foot bath." *Japanese Journal of Medical Mycology* 48, no. 1 (2007): 27–36.

Intahphuak, S., P. Khonsung, and A. Panthong. "Anti-inflammatory, analgesic, and antipyretic activities of virgin coconut oil." *Pharmaceutical biology* 48, no. 2 (2010): 151–157.

Jalali-Heravi, Mehdi, Behrooz Zekavat, and Hassan Sereshti. "Characterization of essential oil components of Iranian geranium oil using gas chromatography–mass spectrometry combined with chemometric resolution techniques." *Journal of Chromatography A* 1114, no. 1 (2006): 154–163.

Johnson, Rebecca L., Steven Foster, Tieraona Low Dog, and David Kiefer *National Geographic Guide to Medicinal Herbs: The World's Most Effective Healing Plants*. National Geographic, 2012.

Kale, Shantanu, Amol Sonawane, Ammar Ansari, Prashant Ghoge, and Ashwini Waje. "Formulation and in-vitro determination of sun protection factor of Ocimum basilicum, Linn. leaf oils sunscreen cream." *Int. J. Pharm. Pharm. Sci*2, no. 4 (2010): 147–149.

Karsha, Pavithra Vani, and O. Bhagya Lakshmi. "Antibacterial activity of black pepper (Piper nigrum Linn.) with special reference to its mode of action on bacteria." *Indian J. Nat. Prod. Resour* 1, no. 2 (2010): 213–215.

Kaur, Chanchal Deep, and Swarnlata Saraf. "In vitro sun protection factor determination of herbal oils used in cosmetics." *Pharmacognosy research* 2, no. 1 (2010): 22.

Kellett, George L., Edith Brot-Laroche, Oliver J. Mace, and Armelle Leturque. "Sugar absorption in the intestine: the role of GLUT2." *Annu. Rev. Nutr.* 28 (2008): 35–54.

Kiecolt-Glaser, Janice K., Jennifer E. Graham, William B. Malarkey, Kyle Porter, Stanley Lemeshow, and Ronald Glaser. "Olfactory influences on mood and autonomic, endocrine, and immune function." *Psychoneuroendocrinology* 33, no. 3 (2008): 328–339.

Kim, H. J., Chen, F., Wang, X., Chung, H. Y., & Jin, Z. (2005). Evaluation of antioxidant activity of vetiver (Vetiveria zizanioides L.) oil and identification of its antioxidant constituents. *Journal of agricultural and food chemistry*, 53(20), 7691–7695.

Kim, Jung T., Michael Wajda, Germaine Cuff, David Serota, Michael Schlame, Deborah M. Axelrod, Amber A. Guth, and Alex Y. Bekker. "Evaluation of aromatherapy in treating postoperative pain: pilot study." *Pain Practice* 6, no. 4 (2006): 273–277.

Kim, Sang Hun, and Hyung Kyou Jun. "Efficacy of aromatherapy for the treatment of otitis externa in dogs." 대한수의학회지 49, no. 1 (2009): 85–89.

Kim, Yong-Guy, Jin-Hyung Lee, Soon-Il Kim, Kwang-Hyun Baek, and Jintae Lee. "Cinnamon bark oil and its components inhibit biofilm formation and toxin production." *International journal of food microbiology* 195 (2015): 30–39.

Kline, Robert M., Jeffrey J. Kline, Joan Di Palma, and Giulio J. Barbero. "Enteric-coated, pH-dependent peppermint oil capsules for the treatment of irritable bowel syndrome in children." *The Journal of pediatrics* 138, no. 1 (2001): 125–128.

Knasko, Susan C. "Ambient odor's effect on creativity, mood, and perceived health." *Chemical Senses* 17, no. 1 (1992): 27–35.

Koči, J., B. Jeffery, J. E. Riviere, and N. A. Monteiro-Riviere. "In vitro safety assessment of food ingredients in canine renal proximal tubule cells."*Toxicology in Vitro* 29, no. 2 (2015): 289–298.

Komiya, Migiwa, Takashi Takeuchi, and Etsumori Harada. "Lemon oil vapor causes an anti-stress effect via modulating the 5-HT and DA activities in mice."*Behavioural Brain Research* 172, no. 2 (2006): 240–249.

Kothiwale, Shaila V., Vivek Patwardhan, Megha Gandhi, Rahul Sohoni, and Ajay Kumar. "A comparative study of antiplaque and antigingivitis effects of herbal mouthrinse containing tea tree oil, clove, and basil with commercially available essential oil mouthrinse." *Journal of Indian Society of Periodontology*18, no. 3 (2014): 316.

Koul, Opender, Suresh Walia, and G. S. Dhaliwal. "Essential oils as green pesticides: potential and constraints." *Biopesticides International* 4, no. 1 (2008): 63–84.

Krishan, Gopal, and Asmita Narang. "Integrative Therapies in Veterinary Practice." *Advanced Journal of Pharmacology and Pharmacotherapeutics* 2, no. 1 (2015): 50–55.

Kristinsson, Karl G., Anna B. Magnusdottir, Hannes Petersen, and Ann Hermansson. "Effective treatment of experimental acute otitis media by application of volatile fluids into the ear canal." *Journal of infectious diseases*191, no. 11 (2005): 1876–1880.

Kwakman, Paulus HS, Johannes PC Van den Akker, Ahmet Güçlü, Hamid Aslami, Jan M. Binnekade, Leonie de Boer, Laura Boszhard et al. "Medical-grade honey kills antibiotic-resistant bacteria in vitro and eradicates skin colonization." *Clinical Infectious Diseases* 46, no. 11 (2008): 1677–1682.

Lad, Vasant. *The complete book of Ayurvedic home remedies*. Harmony, 1999.

Lampl, Christian, Bernhard Haider, and Christine Schweiger. "Long-term efficacy of Boswellia serrata in four patients with chronic cluster headache."*Cephalalgia* 32, no. 9 (2012): 719–722.

Lans, Cheryl, and Kerry Hackett. "Essential oil use in ethnoveterinary medicine in British Columbia, Canada."

Lavania, U. C. "Other uses and utilization of vetiver: vetiver oil." *The Proceedings of the 2003 The Third Int. Conference on Vetiver and Exhibition* (2003) 486–491.

Lee, Jung-Bum, Sachi Miyake, Ryo Umetsu, Kyoko Hayashi, Takeshi Chijimatsu, and Toshimitsu Hayashi. "Anti-influenza A virus effects of fructan from Welsh onion (Allium fistulosum L.)." *Food chemistry* 134, no. 4 (2012): 2164–2168.

Lehrner, Johann, Christine Eckersberger, Peter Walla, G. Pötsch, and Lüder Deecke. "Ambient odor of orange in a dental office reduces anxiety and improves mood in female patients." *Physiology & behavior* 71, no. 1 (2000): 83–86.

Leite, Mariana P., Jaime Fassin Jr, Eliane MF Baziloni, Reinaldo N. Almeida, Rita Mattei, and José R. Leite. "Behavioral effects of essential oil of Citrus aurantium L. inhalation in rats." *Revista Brasileira de Farmacognosia* 18 (2008): 661–666.

Lemenith, M., and D. Teketay. "Frankincense and myrrh resources of Ethiopia: II. Medicinal and industrial uses." *SINET: Ethiopian Journal of Science* 26, no. 2 (2005): 161–172.

Levin, Cheryl, and Howard Maibach. "Exploration of alternative and natural drugs in dermatology." *Archives of dermatology* 138, no. 2 (2002): 207–211.

Lewis, Randine. "Treatment of endometriosis and fibroids with acupuncture."*Acufinder. com* (2013).

Lim, Won Churl, Jeong Min Seo, Chun Il Lee, Hyeong Bae Pyo, and Bum Chun Lee. "Stimulative and sedative effects of essential oils upon inhalation in mice."*Archives of pharmacal research* 28, no. 7 (2005): 770–774.

Lis-Balchin, M., and S. G. Deans. "Bioactivity of selected plant essential oils against Listeria monocytogenes." *Journal of Applied Microbiology* 82, no. 6 (1997): 759–762.

Lupi, Omar, Ivan Jorge Semenovitch, Curt Treu, Daniel Bottino, and Eliete Bouskela. "Evaluation of the effects of caffeine in the microcirculation and edema on thighs and buttocks using the orthogonal polarization spectral imaging and clinical parameters." *Journal of cosmetic dermatology* 6, no. 2 (2007): 102–107.

M Alvarez-Suarez, Jose, Francesca Giampieri, and Maurizio Battino. "Honey as a source of dietary antioxidants: structures, bioavailability and evidence of protective effects against human chronic diseases." *Current medicinal chemistry* 20, no. 5 (2013): 621–638.

Mahmoud, Abeer, Rasha Attia, S. A. I. D. Safaa, and Zedan Ibraheim. "Ginger and Cinnamon: Can This Household Remedy Treat Giardia¬ sis? Parasitological and Histopathological Studies." *Iranian Journal of Parasitology* 9, no. 4 (2014): 530–540.

Mandalari, G., R. N. Bennett, G. Bisignano, D. Trombetta, A. Saija, C. B. Faulds, M. J. Gasson, and A. Narbad. "Antimicrobial activity of flavonoids extracted from bergamot (Citrus bergamia Risso) peel, a byproduct of the essential oil industry." *Journal of Applied Microbiology* 103, no. 6 (2007): 2056–2064.

Mangal, Brijesh, Ayushi Sugandhi, Kanteshwari I. Kumathalli, and Raja Sridhar. "Alternative Medicine in Periodontal Therapy—A Review." *Journal of acupuncture and meridian studies* 5, no. 2 (2012): 51–56.

Marija, Bošković, Baltić Ž. Milan, Ivanović Jelena, Đurić Jelena, Lončina Jasna, Dokmanović Marija, and Marković Radmila. "Use of essential oils in order to prevent food-borne illnesses caused by pathogens in meat." *Tehnologija mesa* 54, no. 1 (2013): 14–20.

Maruyama, Naho, Yuka Sekimoto, Hiroko Ishibashi, Shigeharu Inouye, Haruyuki Oshima, Hideyo Yamaguchi, and Shigeru Abe. "Suppression of neutrophil accumulation in mice by cutaneous application of geranium essential oil." *J inflamm* 2 (2005): 1–11.

McKay, Brett and Kate McKay. *The Art of Manliness* (blog) January 21, 2010 http://www.artofmanliness.com/2010/01/21/diy-bay-rum-aftershave/.

Mead, Paul S., Laurence Slutsker, Vance Dietz, Linda F. McCaig, Joseph S. Bresee, Craig Shapiro, Patricia M. Griffin, and Robert V. Tauxe. "Food-related illness and death in the United States." *Emerging infectious diseases* 5, no. 5 (1999): 607.

Mehmood, Malik Hassan, and Anwarul Hassan Gilani. "Pharmacological basis for the medicinal use of black pepper and piperine in gastrointestinal disorders." *Journal of Medicinal Food* 13, no. 5 (2010): 1086–1096.

Menetrez, Marc Y., Karin K. Foarde, Tricia D. Webber, Timothy R. Dean, and Doris A. Betancourt. "Testing antimicrobial cleaner efficacy on gypsum wallboard contaminated with Stachybotrys chartarum." *Environmental Science and Pollution Research-International* 14, no. 7 (2007): 523–528.

Micol, Vicente, Nuria Caturla, Laura Pérez-Fons, Vicente Más, Luis Pérez, and Amparo Estepa. "The olive leaf extract exhibits antiviral activity against viral haemorrhagic septicaemia rhabdovirus (VHSV)." *Antiviral Research* 66, no. 2 (2005): 129–136.

Mikhaeil, B. R., Maatooq, G. T., Badria, F. A., & Amer, M. M. (2003). Chemistry and immunomodulatory activity of frankincense oil. *Zeitschrift fur Naturforschung C-Journal of Biosciences*, 58(3–4), 230–238.

Milhau, Guilhem, Alexis Valentin, Françoise Benoit, Michèle Mallié, Jean-Marie Bastide, Yves Pélissier, and Jean-Marie Bessière. "In vitro antimalarial activity of eight essential oils." *Journal of Essential Oil Research* 9, no. 3 (1997): 329–333.

Milind, Parle, and Chaturvedi Dev. "Orange: range of benefits." *Int Res J Pharm* 3, no. 7 (2012): 59–63.

Misra, Biswapriya B., and Satyahari Dey. "Evaluation of in vivo anti-hyperglycemic and antioxidant potentials of α-santalol and sandalwood oil."*Phytomedicine* 20, no. 5 (2013): 409–416.

Modern Essentials: A Contemporary Guide to the Therapeutic Use of Essential Oils, Fifth Ed. AromaTools, 2014.

Mojay, Gabriel. *Aromatherapy for healing the spirit: Restoring emotional and mental balance with essential oils.* Inner Traditions/Bear & Co, 2000.

Molan, Peter C. "Why honey is effective as a medicine. 1. Its use in modern medicine." (1999).

Molan, Peter C. "The role of honey in the management of wounds. *Journal of Wound Care* 8, no. 8 (1999), 415–418.

Moore, Eric J., and Eugene B. Kern. "Atrophic rhinitis: a review of 242 cases."*American journal of rhinology* 15, no. 6 (2001): 355–361.

Morris, Neil, Steven Birtwistle, and Margaret Toms. "Anxiety reduction by aromatherapy: anxiolytic effects of inhalation of geranium and rosemary."*International Journal of Aromatherapy* 7, no. 2 (1995): 33–39.

Moss, Mark, Jenny Cook, Keith Wesnes, and Paul Duckett. "Aromas of rosemary and lavender essential oils differentially affect cognition and mood in healthy adults." *International Journal of Neuroscience* 113, no. 1 (2003): 15–38.

Moss, Mark, Steven Hewitt, Lucy Moss, and Keith Wesnes. "Modulation of cognitive performance and mood by aromas of peppermint and ylang-ylang."*International Journal of Neuroscience* 118, no. 1 (2008): 59–77.

Muggli, R. "Systemic evening primrose oil improves the biophysical skin parameters of healthy adults." *International journal of cosmetic science* 27, no. 4 (2005): 243–249.

Nascimento, Gislene GF, Juliana Locatelli, Paulo C. Freitas, and Giuliana L. Silva. "Antibacterial activity of plant extracts and phytochemicals on antibiotic-resistant bacteria." *Brazilian journal of microbiology* 31, no. 4 (2000): 247–256.

Nenoff, P., U-F. Haustein, and W. Brandt. "Antifungal activity of the essential oil of Melaleuca alternifolia (tea tree oil) against pathogenic fungi in vitro." *Skin Pharmacology and Physiology* 9, no. 6 (1996): 388–394.

Ni, Cheng-Hua, Wen-Hsuan Hou, Ching-Chiu Kao, Ming-Li Chang, Lee-Fen Yu, Chia-Che Wu, and Chiehfeng Chen. "The anxiolytic effect of aromatherapy on patients awaiting ambulatory surgery: a randomized controlled trial." *Evidence-Based Complementary and Alternative Medicine* 2013 (2013).

Norrish, Mark Ian Keith, and Katie Louise Dwyer. "Preliminary investigation of the effect of peppermint oil on an objective measure of daytime sleepiness." *International journal of psychophysiology* 55, no. 3 (2005): 291–298.

Ogbazghi, Woldeselassie, F. J. J. M. Bongers, Toon Rijkers, and Marius Wessel. "Population structure and morphology of the frankincense tree Boswellia papyrifera along an altitude gradient in Eritrea." *Journal of the Drylands* 1, no. 1 (2006): 85–94.

Ogbolu, D. O., A. A. Oni, O. A. Daini, and A. P. Oloko. "In vitro antimicrobial properties of coconut oil on Candida species in Ibadan, Nigeria." *Journal of medicinal food* 10, no. 2 (2007): 384–387.

Oliveira, Julyana de Araújo, Ingrid Carla Guedes da Silva, Leonardo Antunes Trindade, Edeltrudes Oliveira Lima, Hugo Lemes Carlo, Alessandro Leite Cavalcanti, and Ricardo Dias de Castro. "Safety and Tolerability of Essential Oil from Cinnamomum zeylanicum Blume Leaves with Action on Oral Candidosis and Its Effect on the Physical Properties of the Acrylic Resin." *Evidence-Based Complementary and Alternative Medicine* 2014 (2014).

Olson, Wanda, Marilyn Bode, and Polly Dubbel. "Hard Surface Cleaning Performance of Six Alternative Household Cleaners Under Laboratory Conditions." Journal of Environmental Health 56, no. 6, (1994) 27–31.

Olukemi, Odukoya A., Jenkins M. Oluseyi, Ilori O. Olukemi, and Sofidiya M. Olutoyin. "The use of selected Nigerian natural products in management of environmentally induced free radical skin damage." *Pakistan Journal of Biological Sciences* 8, no. 8 (2005): 1074–1077.

Omidbaigi, R., F. Sefidkon, and F. Kazemi. "Influence of drying methods on the essential oil content and composition of Roman chamomile." *Flavour and fragrance journal* 19, no. 3 (2004): 196–198.

Omura, Yoshiaki, Nobuko Horiuchi, Marilyn K. Jones, Dominic P. Lu, Yasuhiro Shimotsuura, Harsha Duvvi, Andrew Pallos, Motomu Ohki, and Akihiro Suetsugu. "Temporary Anti-Cancer & Anti-Pain Effects of Mechanical Stimulation of Any One of 3 Front Teeth (1st Incisor, 2nd Incisor, & Canine) of Right & Left Side of Upper & Lower Jaws and Their Possible Mechanism, & Relatively Long Term Disappearance of Pain & Cancer Parameters by One Optimal Dose of DHEA, Astragalus, Boswellia Serrata, often with Press Needle Stimulation of True ST. 36." *Acupuncture & electro-therapeutics research* 34, no. 3–4 (2009): 175–203.

Onawunmi, Grace O., Wolde-Ab Yisak, and E. O. Ogunlana. "Antibacterial constituents in the essential oil of Cymbopogon citratus (DC.) Stapf." *Journal of Ethnopharmacology* 12, no. 3 (1984): 279–286.

Onyeagba, R. A., Ugbogu, O. C., Okeke, C. U., & Iroakasi, O. (2005). Studies on the antimicrobial effects of garlic (Allium sativum Linn), ginger (Zingiber officinale Roscoe) and lime (Citrus aurantifolia Linn). *African Journal of Biotechnology*, 3(10), 552–554.

Ostad, S. N., M. Soodi, M. Shariffzadeh, N. Khorshidi, and H. Marzban. "The effect of fennel essential oil on uterine contraction as a model for dysmenorrhea, pharmacology and toxicology study." *Journal of Ethnopharmacology* 76, no. 3 (2001): 299–304.

Ou, Ming-Chiu, Yu-Fei Lee, Chih-Ching Li, and Shyi-Kuen Wu. "The Effectiveness of Essential Oils for Patients with Neck Pain: A Randomized Controlled Study." *The Journal of Alternative and Complementary Medicine* 20, no. 10 (2014): 771–779.

Ou, Ming Chiu, Tsung Fu Hsu, Andrew C. Lai, Yu Ting Lin, and Chia Ching Lin. "Pain relief assessment by aromatic essential oil massage on outpatients with primary dysmenorrhea: A randomized, double-blind clinical trial." *Journal of Obstetrics and Gynaecology Research* 38, no. 5 (2012): 817–822.

Palazzolo, Eristanna, Vito Armando Laudicina, and Maria Antonietta Germanà. "Current and potential use of citrus essential oils." *Current Organic Chemistry* 17, no. 24 (2013): 3042–3049.

Palombo, Enzo A. "Phytochemicals from traditional medicinal plants used in the treatment of diarrhoea: modes of action and effects on intestinal function." *Phytotherapy Research* 20, no. 9 (2006): 717–724.

Panella, Nicholas A., Joseph Karchesy, Gary O. Maupin, Johannes CS Malan, and Joseph Piesman. "Susceptibility of immature Ixodes scapularis (Acari: Ixodidae) to plant-derived acaricides." *Journal of medical entomology* 34, no. 3 (1997): 340–345.

Patil, Umesh K., Amrit Singh, and Anup K. Chakraborty. "Role of piperine as a bioavailability enhancer." *International Journal of Recent Advances in Pharmaceutical Research* 4 (2011): 16–23.

Pattnaik, S., V. R. Subramanyam, and C. Kole. "Antibacterial and antifungal activity of ten essential oils in vitro." *Microbios* 86 (1996): 237–246.

Peana, Alessandra Tiziana, Paolo Stefano D'Aquila, Francesca Panin, Gino Serra, P. Pippia, and Mario Domenico Luigi Moretti. "Anti-inflammatory activity of linalool and linalyl acetate constituents of essential oils." *Phytomedicine* 9, no. 8 (2002): 721–726.

Peng, Shu-Ming, Malcolm Koo, and Zer-Ran Yu. "Effects of music and essential oil inhalation on cardiac autonomic balance in healthy individuals." *The Journal of alternative and complementary medicine* 15, no. 1 (2009): 53–57.

Pengelly, Andrew, James Snow, Simon Y. Mills, Andrew Scholey, Keith Wesnes, and Leah Reeves Butler. "Short-term study on the effects of rosemary on cognitive function in an elderly population." *Journal of medicinal food* 15, no. 1 (2012): 10–17.

Pichersky, Eran, and David R. Gang. "Genetics and biochemistry of secondary metabolites in plants: an evolutionary perspective." *Trends in plant science* 5, no. 10 (2000): 439–445.

Pinto, Eugénia, Luís Vale-Silva, Carlos Cavaleiro, and Lígia Salgueiro. "Antifungal activity of the clove essential oil from Syzygium aromaticum on Candida, Aspergillus and dermatophyte species." *Journal of Medical Microbiology* 58, no. 11 (2009): 1454–1462.

Poeckel, Daniel, and Oliver Werz. "Boswellic acids: biological actions and molecular targets." *Current medicinal chemistry* 13, no. 28 (2006): 3359–3369.

Politeo, Olivera, M. Jukic, and M. Milos. "Chemical composition and antioxidant capacity of free volatile aglycones from basil (Ocimum basilicum L.) compared with its essential oil." *Food Chemistry* 101, no. 1 (2007): 379–385.

Prabuseenivasan, Seenivasan, Manickkam Jayakumar, and Savarimuthu Ignacimuthu. "In vitro antibacterial activity of some plant essential oils." *BMC complementary and alternative medicine* 6, no. 1 (2006): 39.

Price, Shirley, and Len Price, eds. *Aromatherapy for health professionals.* Elsevier Health Sciences, 2007.

Ransaw, Theodore, ed. *Sexual Secrets of Cleopatra: The Wisdom of the Ancient Egyptians.* iUniverse, 2000.

Rasch, Björn, Christian Büchel, Steffen Gais, and Jan Born. "Odor cues during slow-wave sleep prompt declarative memory consolidation." *Science* 315, no. 5817 (2007): 1426–1429.

Rawlings, A. V. "Cellulite and its treatment." *International journal of cosmetic science* 28, no. 3 (2006): 175–190.

Reddy, G. Kesava, Gowri Chandrakasan, and S. C. Dhar. "Studies on the metabolism of glycosaminoglycans under the influence of new herbal anti-inflammatory agents." *Biochemical pharmacology* 38, no. 20 (1989): 3527–3534.

Reichling, Juergen, Paul Schnitzler, Ulrike Suschke, and Reinhard Saller. "Essential oils of aromatic plants with antibacterial, antifungal, antiviral, and cytotoxic properties-an overview." *Forschende Komplementrmedizin (2006.)* 16, no. 2 (2009): 79.

Reuter, Juliane, Irmgard Merfort, and Christoph M. Schempp. "Botanicals in dermatology." *American journal of clinical dermatology* 11, no. 4 (2010): 247–267.

Rim, In-Sook, and Cha-Ho Jee. "Acaricidal effects of herb essential oils against Dermatophagoides farinae and D. pteronyssinus (Acari: Pyroglyphidae) and qualitative analysis of a herb Mentha pulegium (pennyroyal)." *The Korean journal of parasitology* 44, no. 2 (2006): 133–138.

Roby, Mohamed Hussein Hamdy, Mohamed Atef Sarhan, Khaled Abdel-Hamed Selim, and Khalel Ibrahim Khalel. "Antioxidant and antimicrobial activities of essential oil and extracts of fennel (Foeniculum vulgare L.) and chamomile (Matricaria chamomilla L.)." *Industrial Crops and Products* 44 (2013): 437–445.

Rohloff, Jens. "Monoterpene composition of essential oil from peppermint (Mentha× piperita L.) with regard to leaf position using solid-phase microextraction and gas chromatography/mass spectrometry analysis." *Journal of agricultural and food chemistry* 47, no. 9 (1999): 3782–3786.

Rozza, Ariane Leite, Thiago de Mello Moraes, Hélio Kushima, Alexandre Tanimoto, Márcia Ortiz Mayo Marques, Taís Maria Bauab, Clélia Akiko Hiruma-Lima, and Cláudia Helena Pellizzon. "Gastroprotective mechanisms of Citrus lemon (Rutaceae) essential oil and its majority compounds limonene and β-pinene: involvement of heat-shock protein-70, vasoactive intestinal peptide, glutathione, sulfhydryl compounds, nitric oxide and prostaglandin E 2." *Chemico-biological interactions* 189, no. 1 (2011): 82–89.

Saarinen, K., J. Jantunen, and T. Haahtela. "Birch pollen honey for birch pollen allergy–A randomized controlled pilot study." *International archives of allergy and immunology* 155, no. 2 (2011): 160–166.

Saeki, Y. "The effect of foot-bath with or without the essential oil of lavender on the autonomic nervous system: a randomized trial." *Complementary Therapies in Medicine* 8, no. 1 (2000): 2–7.

Safayhi, H., and E. R. Sailer. "Anti-inflammatory actions of pentacyclic triterpenes." *Planta medica* 63, no. 6 (1997): 487–493.

Saleem, TS Mohamed, S. Darbar Basha, G. Mahesh, PV Sandhya Rani, N. Suresh Kumar, and C. M. Chetty. "Analgesic, anti-pyretic and anti-inflammatory activity of dietary sesame oil in experimental animal models." *Pharmacologia* 2, no. 6 (2011): 172–177.

Sandoval-Montemayor, Nallely E., Abraham García, Elizabeth Elizondo-Treviño, Elvira Garza-González, Laura Alvarez, and María del Rayo Camacho-Corona. "Chemical composition of hexane extract of Citrus aurantifolia and anti-Mycobacterium tuberculosis activity of some of its constituents." *Molecules* 17, no. 9 (2012): 11173–11184.

Santoro, G. F., M. G. Cardoso, L. G. L. Guimarães, J. M. Freire, and M. J. Soares. "Anti-proliferative effect of the essential oil of Cymbopogon citratus (DC) Stapf (lemongrass) on intracellular amastigotes, bloodstream trypomastigotes and culture epimastigotes of Trypanosoma cruzi (Protozoa: Kinetoplastida)." *Parasitology* 134, no. 11 (2007): 1649–1656.

Santoyo, S., S. Cavero, L. Jaime, E. Ibanez, F. J. Senorans, and G. Reglero. "Chemical composition and antimicrobial activity of Rosmarinus officinalis L. essential oil obtained via supercritical fluid extraction." *Journal of Food Protection®* 68, no. 4 (2005): 790–795.

Sarrell, E. Michael, Herman Avner Cohen, and Ernesto Kahan. "Naturopathic treatment for ear pain in children." *Pediatrics* 111, no. 5 (2003): e574-e579.

Sasannejad, Payam, Morteza Saeedi, Ali Shoeibi, Ali Gorji, Maryam Abbasi, and Mohsen Foroughipour. "Lavender essential oil in the treatment of migraine headache: a placebo-controlled clinical trial." *European neurology* 67 (2012): 288–91.

Satchell, Andrew C., Anne Saurajen, Craig Bell, and Ross StC Barnetson. "Treatment of interdigital tinea pedis with 25% and 50% tea tree oil solution: A randomized, placebo-controlled, blinded study." *Australasian journal of dermatology* 43, no. 3 (2002): 175–178.

Schnaubelt, Kurt. *The healing intelligence of essential oils: the science of advanced aromatherapy.* Inner Traditions/Bear & Co, 2011.

Schneider, Rainer. "There Is Something in the Air: Testing the Efficacy of a new Olfactory Stress Relief Method (AromaStick®)." *Stress and Health* (2015).

Seo, Ji-Yeong. "The effects of aromatherapy on stress and stress responses in adolescents." *Journal of Korean Academy of Nursing* 39, no. 3 (2009): 357–365.

Seol, Geun Hee, Hyun Soo Shim, Pill-Joo Kim, Hea Kyung Moon, Ki Ho Lee, Insop Shim, Suk Hyo Suh, and Sun Seek Min. "Antidepressant-like effect of Salvia sclarea is explained by modulation of dopamine activities in rats." *Journal of ethnopharmacology* 130, no. 1 (2010): 187–190.

Shi, John, Jianmel Yu, Joseph E. Pohorly, and Yukio Kakuda. "Polyphenolics in grape seeds-biochemistry and functionality." *Journal of medicinal food* 6, no. 4 (2003): 291–299.

Shin, S., and S. Lim. "Antifungal effects of herbal essential oils alone and in combination with ketoconazole against Trichophyton spp." *Journal of applied microbiology* 97, no. 6 (2004): 1289–1296.

Shin, Seungwon. "Anti-Aspergillus activities of plant essential oils and their combination effects with ketoconazole or amphotericin B." *Archives of pharmacal research* 26, no. 5 (2003): 389–393.

Silva, Jeane, Worku Abebe, S. M. Sousa, V. G. Duarte, M. I. L. Machado, and F. J. A. Matos. "Analgesic and anti-inflammatory effects of essential oils of Eucalyptus." *Journal of ethnopharmacology* 89, no. 2 (2003): 277–283.

Singh, Ramnik, Narinder Singh, B. S. Saini, and Harwinder Singh Rao. "In vitro antioxidant activity of pet ether extract of black pepper." *Indian journal of pharmacology* 40, no. 4 (2008): 147.

Smith-Palmer, A., J. Stewart, and Lorna Fyfe. "Antimicrobial properties of plant essential oils and essences against five important food-borne pathogens."*Letters in applied microbiology* 26, no. 2 (1998): 118–122.

Soh, Melissa, and Gwidon W. Stachowiak. "The application of cineole as a grease solvent." *Flavour and fragrance journal* 17, no. 4 (2002): 278–286.

Soltani, R., Soheilipour, S., Hajhashemi, V., Asghari, G., Bagheri, M., & Molavi, M. (2013). Evaluation of the effect of aromatherapy with lavender essential oil on post-tonsillectomy pain in pediatric patients: a randomized controlled trial.*International journal of pediatric otorhinolaryngology*, 77(9), 1579–1581.

Srinivasan, Krishnapura. "Spices as influencers of body metabolism: an overview of three decades of research." *Food Research International* 38, no. 1 (2005): 77–86.

Srivastava, Janmejai K., and Sanjay Gupta. "Health promoting benefits of chamomile in the elderly population." *Complementary and Alternative Therapies in the Aging Population* (2011): 135.

Srivastava, Janmejai K., Eswar Shankar, and Sanjay Gupta. "Chamomile: A herbal medicine of the past with a bright future (Review)." *Molecular medicine reports* 3, no. 6 (2010): 895–901.

STAPPEN, I., M. HÖFERL, and E. HEUBERGER. "Behavioral and Endocrine Effects of Essential Oils in Humans." *Sci Pharm* 77 (2009): 185.

Sutoh, Madoka, Shuichi Ito, Etsuko Kasuya, and Ken-ichi YAYOU. "Effects of exposure to plant-derived odorants on behavior and the concentration of stress-related hormones in steers isolated under a novel environment." *Animal Science Journal* 84, no. 2 (2013): 159–164.

Takaki, I., L. E. Bersani-Amado, A. Vendruscolo, S. M. Sartoretto, S. P. Diniz, C. A. Bersani-Amado, and R. K. N. Cuman. "Anti-inflammatory and antinociceptive effects of Rosmarinus officinalis L. essential oil in experimental animal models." *Journal of medicinal food* 11, no. 4 (2008): 741–746.

Takeda, Hitomi, Junzo Tsujita, Mitsuharu Kaya, Masanori Takemura, and Yoshitaka Oku. "Differences between the physiologic and psychologic effects of aromatherapy body treatment." *The Journal of Alternative and Complementary Medicine* 14, no. 6 (2008): 655–661.

Tangpu V, Yadav TA. "Some Important Folklore Medicinal Plants Used by Tangkhul Nagas of Ukhrul District, Manipur." *Recent Progress in Medicinal Plants* 16 (2006): 311–322.

Tao, Neng-guo, Yue-jin Liu, and Miao-ling Zhang. "Chemical composition and antimicrobial activities of essential oil from the peel of bingtang sweet orange (Citrus sinensis Osbeck)." *International journal of food science & technology* 44, no. 7 (2009): 1281–1285.

Thubthimthed, Sirinan, Krittiya Thisayakorn, Ubon Rerk-am, Sinn Tangstirapakdee, and Taweesak Suntorntanasat. "Vetiver oil and its sedative effect." *Thailand Institute of Scientific and Technological Research. ICV3-Proceedings* (2003).

Tiainen, Blanka. "Using aromatherapy and hydrotherapy in obstetrics care–study on labouring womens perceptions." *University Of Eastern Finland* (2014): 1–59.

Tillett, Jackie, and Diane Ames. "The uses of aromatherapy in women's health." *The Journal of perinatal & neonatal nursing* 24, no. 3 (2010): 238–245.

Tisserand, Robert, and Rodney Young. *Essential oil safety: a guide for health care professionals*. Elsevier Health Sciences, 2013.

Tisserand, Robert. "Essential oils as psychotherapeutic agents." In *Perfumery*, pp. 167–181. Springer Netherlands, 1988.

Tisserand, Robert. *The art of aromatherapy: The healing and beautifying properties of the essential oils of flowers and herbs*. Inner Traditions/Bear & Co, 1977.

Torii, Shizuo. "Odour mechanisms: The psychological benefits of odours." *International Journal of Aromatherapy* 8, no. 3 (1997): 34–39.

Tripathi, Arun K., Shikha Upadhyay, Mantu Bhuiyan, and P. R. Bhattacharya. "A review on prospects of essential oils as biopesticide in insect-pest management." *Journal of Pharmacognosy and Phytotherapy* 1, no. 5 (2009): 52–63.

Tripoli, Elisa, Marco Giammanco, Garden Tabacchi, Danila Di Majo, Santo Giammanco, and Maurizio La Guardia. "The phenolic compounds of olive oil: structure, biological activity and beneficial effects on human health." *Nutrition Research Reviews* 18, no. 01 (2005): 98–112.

Troisi, Jordan D., and Shira Gabriel. "Chicken Soup Really Is Good for the Soul "Comfort Food" Fulfills the Need to Belong." *Psychological Science* 22, no. 6 (2011): 747–753.

Trumble, John T. "Caveat emptor: safety considerations for natural products used in arthropod control." *AMERICAN ENTOMOLOGIST-LANHAM-* 48, no. 1 (2002): 7–13.

Tung, Yu-Tang, Meng-Thong Chua, Sheng-Yang Wang, and Shang-Tzen Chang. "Anti-inflammation activities of essential oil and its constituents from indigenous cinnamon (Cinnamomum osmophloeum) twigs." *Bioresource Technology* 99, no. 9 (2008): 3908–3913.

Turner Jr, John, Anna DeLeon, Cathy Gibson, and Thomas Fine. "Effects of Flotation REST on Range of Motion, Grip Strength and Pain in Rheumatoid Arthritics." In *Clinical and Experimental Restricted Environmental Stimulation*, pp. 297–306. Springer New York, 1993.

Tzortzakis, Nikos G., and Costas D. Economakis. "Antifungal activity of lemongrass (Cympopogon citratus L.) essential oil against key postharvest pathogens." *Innovative Food Science & Emerging Technologies* 8, no. 2 (2007): 253–258.

Umezu, Toyoshi, Akiko Sakata, and Hiroyasu Ito. "Ambulation-promoting effect of peppermint oil and identification of its active constituents." *Pharmacology Biochemistry and Behavior* 69, no. 3 (2001): 383–390.

Umezu, Toyoshi. "Evidence for dopamine involvement in ambulation promoted by menthone in mice." *Pharmacology Biochemistry and Behavior* 91, no. 3 (2009): 315–320.

Urbaniak, A., A. Głowacka, E. Kowalczyk, M. Lysakowska, and M. Sienkiewicz. "[The antibacterial activity of cinnamon oil on the selected gram-positive and gram-negative bacteria]." *Medycyna doswiadczalna i mikrobiologia* 66, no. 2 (2013): 131–141.

Vakilian, Katayon, and Afsaneh Keramat. "The Effect of the Breathing Technique With and Without Aromatherapy on the Length of the Active Phase and Second Stage of Labor." *Nursing and midwifery studies* 1, no. 3 (2013): 115–119.

Van Vuuren, S. F., G. P. P. Kamatou, and A. M. Viljoen. "Volatile composition and antimicrobial activity of twenty commercial frankincense essential oil samples." *South African Journal of Botany* 76, no. 4 (2010): 686–691.

Vendruscolo, A., I. Takaki, L. E. Bersani-Amado, J. A. Dantas, C. A. Bersani-Amado, and R. K. Cuman. "Antiinflammatory and antinociceptive activities of zingiber officinale roscoe essential oil in experimental animal models." *Indian journal of pharmacology* 38, no. 1 (2006): 58.

Verma, Nandini, Rina Chakrabarti, Rakha H. Das, and Hemant K. Gautam. "Anti-inflammatory effects of shea butter through inhibition of iNOS, COX-2, and cytokines via the Nf-Kb pathway in Lps-activated J774 macrophage cells." *Journal of Complementary and Integrative Medicine* 9, no. 1 (2012): 1–11.

Verzera, A., A. Trozzi, G. Dugo, G. Di Bella, and A. Cotroneo. "Biological lemon and sweet orange essential oil composition." *Flavour and fragrance journal* 19, no. 6 (2004): 544–548.

Villar, David, M. J. Knight, S. R. Hansen, and W. B. Buck. "Toxicity of melaleuca oil and related essential oils applied topically on dogs and cats." *Veterinary and human toxicology* 36, no. 2 (1994): 139–142.

Viña, Amparo, and Elizabeth Murillo. "Essential oil composition from twelve varieties of basil (Ocimum spp) grown in Colombia." *Journal of the Brazilian Chemical Society* 14, no. 5 (2003): 744–749.

Visioli, Francesco, and Claudio Galli. "Olive oil phenols and their potential effects on human health." *Journal of Agricultural and Food Chemistry* 46, no. 10 (1998): 4292–4296.

Viuda-Martos, M., Y. Ruiz-Navajas, J. Fernández-López, and J. Pérez-Álvarez. "Antifungal activity of lemon (Citrus lemon L.), mandarin (Citrus reticulata L.), grapefruit (Citrus paradisi L.) and orange (Citrus sinensis L.) essential oils."*Food control* 19, no. 12 (2008): 1130–1138.

Walla, Peter, Bernd Hufnagl, Johann Lehrner, Dagmar Mayer, Gerald Lindinger, Herwig Imhof, Lüder Deecke, and Wilfried Lang. "Olfaction and depth of word processing: a magnetoencephalographic study." *Neuroimage* 18, no. 1 (2003): 104–116.

Warnke, Patrick H., Stephan T. Becker, Rainer Podschun, Sureshan Sivananthan, Ingo N. Springer, Paul AJ Russo, Joerg Wiltfang, Helmut Fickenscher, and Eugene Sherry. "The battle against multi-resistant strains: renaissance of antimicrobial essential oils as a promising force to fight hospital-acquired infections." *Journal of Cranio-Maxillofacial Surgery* 37, no. 7 (2009): 392–397.

Watt, Gillian van der, and Aleksandar Janca. "Aromatherapy in nursing and mental health care." *Contemporary Nurse* 30, no. 1 (2008): 69–75.

Wells, Deborah L. "Aromatherapy for travel-induced excitement in dogs." *Journal of the American Veterinary Medical Association* 229, no. 6 (2006): 964–967.

Wenk, Caspar. "Herbs and botanicals as feed additives in monogastric animals." *Asian Australasian Journal of Animal Sciences* 16, no. 2 (2003): 282–289.

Wheatley, David. "Medicinal plants for insomnia: a review of their pharmacology, efficacy and tolerability." *Journal of psychopharmacology* 19.4 (2005): 414–421.

Williams, Wendy. "Preconception care and aromatherapy in pregnancy." *International Journal of Clinical Aromatherapy* 2, no. 1 (2005) 15–19.

Woelk, H., and S. Schläfke. "A multi-center, double-blind, randomised study of the Lavender oil preparation Silexan in comparison to Lorazepam for generalized anxiety disorder." *Phytomedicine* 17, no. 2 (2010): 94–99.

Wojciechowska, Katarzyna, Maria Zun, Dorota Dwornicka, Katarzyna Swiader, Regina Kasperek, and Ewa Poleszak. "Physical properties and caffeine release from creams prepared with different oils." *Current Issues in Pharmacy and Medical Sciences* 27, no. 4 (2014): 224–228.

Worwood, Valerie Ann. *The Complete Book of Essential Oils and Aromatherapy: Over 600 Natural, Non-toxic & Fragrant Recipes to Create Health• Beauty• A Safe Home Environment.* New World Library, 2012.

Yang, Young-Cheol, Hoi-Seon Lee, J. M. Clark, and Young-Joon Ahn. "Insecticidal activity of plant essential oils against Pediculus humanus capitis (Anoplura: Pediculidae)." *Journal of medical entomology* 41, no. 4 (2004): 699–704.

Yip, Yin Bing, and Ada Chung Ying Tam. "An experimental study on the effectiveness of massage with aromatic ginger and orange essential oil for moderate-to-severe knee pain among the elderly in Hong Kong."*Complementary therapies in medicine* 16, no. 3 (2008): 131–138.

Yoon, Sungpil, Jooheung Lee, and Seungchul Lee. "The therapeutic effect of evening primrose oil in atopic dermatitis patients with dry scaly skin lesions is associated with the normalization of serum gamma-interferon levels." *Skin Pharmacology and Physiology* 15, no. 1 (2002): 20–25.

Yun, Juan, Xuetong Fan, Xihong Li, Tony Z. Jin, Xiaoyu Jia, and James P. Mattheis. "Natural surface coating to inactivate Salmonella enterica serovar Typhimurium and maintain quality of cherry tomatoes." *International journal of food microbiology* 193 (2015): 59–67.

Index

Coconut oil, 11, 25, 26, 29, 39, 40, 42, 43, 50, 86, 87, 90, 91, 97, 98, 99, 132, 133, 136, 142, 143, 152, 153, 154, 155, 160
Comforting diaper cream, 86
Common cold, 19
Conditioning hair rinse, 137
Constipation relief capsule, 52
Constipation relief massage blend, 52
Constipation relief protocol, 51–53
Constipation relief reflexology blend, 53
Constipation relief tea, 52
Cooling sunscreen, 132
Cornstarch, 86, 87, 150
Creativity boosting diffuser blend, 69
Cut, scrape, and burn salve, 42
Cypress essential oil, 20, 22, 78, 81, 97, 98, 99, 126, 127

D

Dandruff protocol, 138
Detoxifying blend, 57
Diarrhea calming capsule, 50
Diarrhea calming massage blend, 50
Diarrhea calming tea, 49
Diarrhea protocol, 49–51
Dog flea spray, 101
Dusting spray, 170

E

Earache relief protocol, 99
Eczema lotion bar, 130
Enterococcus faecalis, 161, 163
Escherichia coli, 46, 47, 48, 97, 161, 163
Essential oils
  aromatic use of, 10–11
  benefits of, 4
  description of, 3–4
  diffusers, 10
  functions, 3
  internal use of, 11
  quality of, 11–13
  reasons for using, 4–5
  safety of, 13–14
  storage of, 15
  topical use of, 11
Eucalyptus essential oil, 28, 30, 31, 32, 66, 68, 104, 140, 141, 164
Evening flower bodywash, 111
Evening primrose oil, 11, 130, 131, 147

F

Fennel essential oil, 39, 40, 50, 51, 52, 53, 57, 60
Fertility support protocol, 74–82
Flu bomb protocol, 19–22
Flu fighting foot rub, 21
Flu fighting gargle, 20
Flu fighting neck and chest rub, 20
Food poisoning prevention capsule, 46
Frankincense (Boswellia species) essential oil, 8, 25, 26, 35, 36, 37, 38, 41, 42, 43, 61, 62, 64, 65, 69, 70, 75, 76, 81, 83, 84, 88, 89, 92, 94, 95, 118, 119, 124, 125, 131, 132, 133, 134, 135, 150, 151

G

Garlic, 21, 22, 48
Gentle rosemary-orange shampoo, 135
Geranium essential oil, 31, 32, 39, 40, 69, 70, 76, 77, 81, 82, 83, 84, 93, 95, 96, 144, 147, 148, 149, 165, 166, 167
Giardia, 48
Giardia lamblia, 46, 47
Ginger essential oil, 27, 39, 40, 41, 48, 49, 50, 52, 54, 57, 60, 75, 81, 145, 146
Glycerin, 85, 86, 95, 96, 97, 109, 110, 111, 112, 117, 118, 119, 120, 123
Grapefruit essential oil, 69, 70, 75, 76, 81, 90, 92, 116, 124, 145, 146, 156, 171, 174
Grape-seed oil, 82, 132, 133
Green onions, 27
Green tea bags, 134
Gunk- and grease-removing spray, 164

H

Hangover relief protocol, 56–60
Hay fever relief diffuser blend, 33
Hay fever relief protocol, 32–34
Headache temple rub, 36
Head cold tea, 26
Healthy nail oil, 152
Himalayan crystal salts, 147, 148, 149, 150
Honey, 19, 24, 25, 33, 42, 43, 45, 48, 49, 55, 56, 75, 81, 113, 114, 122, 140, 141
"Hot" oils, 13, 27, 54

I

Ingestible hay fever relief, 33
Invigorating, cellulite-reducing salt scrub, 145

Proteus vulgaris, 96
Pseudomonas aeruginosa, 48, 97, 161, 163

R
Raw sugar, 142, 143
Refined sugar, 143, 144
Restful wash, 118
Roman chamomile (Chamaemelum nobile
  a.k.a. Anthemis nobilis) essential oil, 7,
  25, 26, 32, 36, 39, 41, 42, 43, 44, 82, 83,
  84, 85, 86, 87, 88, 93, 102, 103, 111, 112,
  128, 129, 131, 132, 134, 135, 139, 149,
  153, 154
Romantic massage blend, 70
Rosemary (Rosmarinus officinalis) essential
  oil, 9, 20, 22, 23, 31, 32, 35, 36, 43, 44,
  52, 53, 54, 57, 59, 60, 66, 67, 68, 104,
  117, 118, 124, 125, 135, 136, 137, 139,
  145, 146, 156

S
Salmonella, 46, 47
Salmonella enterica, 161, 163
Salmonella typhi, 48
Sandalwood essential oil, 64, 65, 71, 73, 88,
  89, 92, 93, 120, 121, 122, 124, 125, 126,
  127, 137, 138, 144, 149
Sanitizing counter spray, 160
Secondary metabolites, 3
Serene shaving cream, 112
Serene soak bath salts, 148
Serratia marcescens, 161, 163
Sesame oil, 41
Shea butter, 112, 113, 120, 122, 128, 129,
  130, 131
Shower steamers, 28
Sinusitis rinse, 30
Sleepy time foot massage blend, 93
Smoothing foot scrub, 153
Soothing foot soak, 153
Sore throat gargle, 24
Soup enhancer, 21
Sparking glass cleaner, 169
SPF level, 132, 133, 134
Staphylococcus, 46
Staphylococcus aureus, 48, 97, 161, 163
Sting and bite compress, 43
Stomach bug bomb, 47
Streptococcus faecalis, 48

Stress-relieving diffuser blend, 63
Study time diffuser blend, 66
Sweet almond oil, 11, 20, 37, 39, 50, 57, 59,
  61, 63, 71, 73, 93, 113, 120, 124, 125,
  126, 144, 147, 160
Sweet and subtle sugar scrub, 143

T
Tantrum taming base, 88
Tantrum taming diffuser blend, 89
Tantrum taming massage blend, 90
Tantrum taming protocol, 88–92
Tantrum taming sensory dough, 91
Terpenes, 3
Thyme essential oil, 46, 47, 57, 60, 77, 80
Trypanosoma, 48

U
Uterine support massage blend, 76

V
Vapor rub, 29
Vegetable capsule, 45, 46, 50, 52, 55
Vetiver essential oil, 64, 65, 69, 70, 88, 89, 91,
  92, 118, 119, 120, 124, 125, 128, 129
Vitamin E oil, 136

W
Wake-up wash, 117
Warm and woody shaving cream, 120
West Indian bay essential oil, 122, 123, 124,
  125, 126, 127
White fir essential oil, 159, 162
White vinegar, 159, 160, 161, 169
Winter diffuser blend, 22, 23
Witch hazel, 94, 95, 96
Woodland cream deodorant, 126

Y
Ylang-ylang essential oil, 64, 65, 71, 72, 76,
  77, 81, 83, 84, 88, 89, 92, 111, 112, 113,
  114, 137, 138, 143, 144, 148, 149, 171,
  172